Guideline for Applied Hygi
2nd revised a

Composition of the working group 2005

Members of the working group and task groups 2005 (in alphabetical order)
Alvensleben, Dr. Braunwarth, Brosinsky, Dr. Bundschu, Dr. Detemple, Dopplé, Fenselau, Frei, Prof. Dr. Frösner, Gorke, Hein, Heisler, Heller, Hofstätter, Hohenadel, Karle, Kief, Prof. Dr. Köhler, Prof. Dr. Kramer, Dr. Krietemeyer, Küntzle, Lamprecht, Dr. Lohmeyer, Dr. Materna, Dr. Mergeryan, Niehus, Dr. Nystrand, Pohl, Schamp, Dr. Schaule, Sommer, Spindler, Tast , Thienel

Institutions of the members 2005 (in alphabetical order)
AfnP, Arbeitsgemeinschaft für nephrologisches Pflegepersonal, Bielefeld · Bio-TeQ Nystrand Consulting, Malmö · B. Braun Melsungen AG, Melsungen · DAGKN – Deutsche Arbeitsgemeinschaft für klinische Nephrologie, Fulda · DGKH – Deutsche Gesellschaft für Krankenhaushygiene, Greifswald · Dialysezentrum und nephrologische Praxis, Backnang · DWA GmbH + Co KG, Ubstadt-Weiher · European Dialysis and Transplant Nurses Association/European Renal Care Association, EDTNA/ERCA, Deutscher Zweig, Essen · Fresenius Medical Care Deutschland GmbH, Bad Homburg · Gambro Hospal GmbH, Planegg · GML Gesellschaft für Medizintechnik und Logistikmanagement mbH, Dresden · Ifw – Institut für Fort- und Weiterbildung der PHV, Ludwigsburg · IWW – Rheinisch-Westfälische Institute für Forschung und Beratung im Wasserfach, Mülheim an der Ruhr · KfH – Kuratorium für Dialyse und Nierentransplantation e.V., Neu-Isenburg · Lauer Membran Wassertechnik GmbH, Wittlingen · Max v. Pettenkofer-Institut, Abt. Virologie, München · Mikrobiologisches Labor Dr. J. Balfanz, Dr. M. Lohmeyer, Münster · Nephrolog. Zentrum Niedersachsen der Arbeiterwohlfahrt, Hannoversch-Münden · Nikkiso Medical GmbH, Hamburg · PHV – Der Dialysepartner Patienten-Heimversorgung gemeinnützige Stiftung, Bad Homburg · Phoenix Pure Water Wasseraufbereitung, Ubstadt-Weiher · Schülke & Mayr GmbH, Norderstedt · S-med Medizintechnik GmbH, Greven · Universitätskliniken Göttingen, Betriebseinheit Krankenhaushygiene und Infektionskontrolle, Göttingen · Universitätsklinikum des Saarlandes, Homburg/Saar

Members of Editorial Group (2005)
Dr. Detemple, Gorke, Hofstätter, Kief, Küntzle, Niehus, Pohl, Thienel

Members of Editorial Group 2009 of the English Edition
Dr. Detemple, Gorke, Hofstätter, Kief, Dr. Krietemeyer, Küntzle, Pohl

Translation and Editorial Support 2009
Akin, Gerrish, Kostadinova, Thomas, Wiedenmann

Financial support of Translation Services by
B. Braun Melsungen AG, Melsungen · Fresenius Medical Care Deutschland GmbH, Bad Homburg · Gambro Hospal GmbH, Planegg · Nikkiso Medical GmbH, Hamburg

Address for correspondence
Pabst Science Publishers

Guideline for Applied Hygiene in Dialysis Units

Edited by
Working Group for Applied Hygiene in Dialysis Units

Pabst Science Publishers
Lengerich · Berlin · Bremen · Miami · Riga · Viernheim · Wien · Zagreb

Bibliographic information published by Die Deutsche Nationalbibliothek
Die Deutsche Nationalbibliothek lists this publication in the Deutsche Nationalbibliografie; detailed bibliographic data is available in the Internet at <http://dnb.ddb.de>.

PABST SCIENCE PUBLISHERS · D-49525 Lengerich
Internet: www.pabst-publishers.de
E-mail: pabst@pabst-publishers.de

ISBN: 978-3-89967-577-1

Typesetting: μ
Printing: KM-Druck · D-64823 Groß-Umstadt

Table of Content

Preface to the 2nd Edition

The content of the first edition of the guidelines[1] represents a standard ("Best-practice guidelines") which was worked out by experts of a national multi-professional working group dealing with the subject "Applied Hygiene in Dialysis". Important reason for the publication of the first edition was a deficit of binding statements from manufacturers and distributors dealing with the questions of hygiene during the use of medical devices and a lack of practically orientated descriptions of measures for operators, managers and users in the existing guidelines, regulations and laws.

Due to the developments in Europe, a changed engineering process and alterations in current and future legislation, it makes sense to look at hygienic processes in the second edition under the view points of an already process-orientated quality management system. The goals are to be predetermined according to the requirements, and measures to respect the limit values shall be described. They can be requested by examining bodies and have to be corrected using adequate measures in case of infringements as well as deviations.

The cross-reference to quality management as the basis of hygiene management and the scientific claims of the group requires that the requests mentioned are supported by valid literature citations. As a result, the working group carried out extensive literature research during the revision of this edition.

More than ever before, quality of treatment has to orientate itself towards economic requirements and standards. In the meantime the legislator has placed higher priority on prevention. As a result, investments for the prevention of additional complications and

[1] Leitlinie für die Praxis der angewandten Hygiene in Behandlungseinheiten für Dialyse, Hrsg. Arbeitskreis für angewandte Hygiene in der Dialyse, Pabst Science Publishers, 1998

costs under the aspect of security and efficiency can have a noticeable effect on the current running costs of treatment, care and technical provisions.

The present work is the result of the participation of highly committed experts. The result of this national and multi-professional working group is based on detailed knowledge, long term experience, diversity and the ability to reach consensus. I would like to thank all the members of the working group and the task groups for their excellent collaboration as well as the companies involved for their advice and their financial and technical support.

Alois Gorke
Co-ordinator of the working group

Additional preface to the translated 2nd Edition 2008 in English

A multidisciplinary workgroup in Germany has published two editions of "Guideline for Practical Hygiene in Dialysis Units" in 1998 and 2005.

The workgroup was founded in 1993 and, over the years, has included approx. 35 organisations and 50 co-workers. Both user organisations, doctors, nurses, hygienists, microbiologists, laboratories, producers of dialysis equipment, producers of water systems for dialysis, virologists, producers of disinfectants and nephrologists have participated.

The "Guideline" is covering all aspects of hygiene in dialysis. Since dialysis as such is an universal procedure, the issues of hygiene will be similar regardless of geographical area.

The workgroup wish to spread the knowledge, experience and information in the "guideline", which has been put together.

There are few documents in the field of hygiene which are covering all aspects.

Some references to laws and regulations are directed to German conditions, but these may of course be replaced by applicable local regulations and/or recommendations.

The workgroup is hoping that the English edition of the "Guideline" will prove to be an easily comprehensible and efficient reference for hygiene issues in the daily work in dialysis units.

Dr. Rolf Nystrand

1 Introduction

Treatment units for renal replacement therapy, e.g. various methods of dialysis, are among the areas with possible risk of infection.[2] The immunodeficiency of the dialysis patient, the risk of transmission of infectious diseases (e.g. hepatitis B viruses (HBV), hepatitis C viruses (HCV), human immunodeficiency virus (HIV) and multi-resistant pathogens (MRP)), the high technical demand of the treatment as well as the requirement for a regular repetition of the treatment, all these factors require that a distinct consciousness and behaviour concerning hygiene is respected by all those concerned within the facility.

The working group, called "Arbeitskreis (AK) für angewandte Hygiene in Dialyseeinheiten" ("Working Group for Applied Hygiene in Dialysis Units" in Germany) started work in May 1993. It arose from the obvious need of reproducibility of the disinfection procedures of the various dialysis machines and supply systems. At that time, guidelines and legal instructions as well as the information of the manufacturers of devices and procedures left important unanswered questions about their use in current practise.

The working group collects and discusses the experience and knowledge of hygiene in current practice of dialysis considering international publications, e.g.

- Infektionsschutzgesetz (Infection Protection Act),
- Guidelines for hospital hygiene and prevention of infections of the Robert Koch Institute[3] (RKI),
- Dialysis standard of the German Working Group for Clinical Nephrology[4] (DAGKN),

[2] RKI-Empfehlung: Anforderungen der Hygiene bei Reinigung und Desinfektion von Flächen. Bundesgesundheitsbl – Gesundheitsforsch – Gesundheitsschutz, 2004 (47): 51-61 (www.rki.de)

[3] RKI: www.rki.de

[4] DAGKN: www.nephrologie.de

- Application rules for haemodialysis of the German Commission for Electrical, Electronic & Information Technologies (DKE)[5]

and other European and International standards with the goal to jointly compile practice-oriented and hygiene-conscious guidelines for the work of dialysis staff.

The latest version is always valid when using legal texts and referring to internet addresses. All the internet addresses cited were checked at the time of going to press. Deviations from the text of this guideline and supplements are possible.

1.1 Goals, Structure and Working Method of the Working Group

The working group set itself the general goal of quality assurance and improvement in the field of hygiene in dialysis. At the same time partial goals are to be considered:

- Deepening the knowledge of the users, the companies involved and other professional groups on hygiene in dialysis
- Re-examining the relevance of existing guidelines to the present circumstances and translating them into practice
- Compiling the basics for the education of users
- Putting together recommendations and requirements for the manufacturers of technical installations and dialysis machines as well as consumables
- Developing standards for collecting, examining and evaluating microbiological samples
- Informing the associations and decision-making organs on the expert opinion and adding these to the guidelines
- Adjusting/revising the existing guidelines

[5] DKE: www.dke.de

The participants come from companies, providers of dialysis treatment, nephrological therapy, nursing and care associations, public authorities and other organisations.

Within this circle there are:

- Physicians specialised in nephrology
- Nephrology nurses
- Dialysis technicians
- Hygienists and microbiologists
- Engineers for occupational health and safety, construction, environment and hygiene among others
- Manufacturers and distributors of medical devices (dialysis machines, water treatment plants and dialysis consumables) and disinfectants.

The working group met about 4 times per year till the end of the revision for a new edition of the guideline.

The revision of individual chapters, the discussion and exchange during meetings and in electronic form with up-to-date return took place in sub-committees and results were sent back to the co-ordinator/moderator of the working group who took care that the texts were distributed to all the working group members for comments and discussion during the working group meetings.

Chapters which have already been approved cannot be changed without the approval of a majority of the working group. Propositions for changes will be sent to the co-ordinator of the working group who after consulting the working group can arrange for further action.

The working group named an editorial board which was responsible for the completion of the new edition. Printing and if necessary reprints were and will be ordered by the co-ordinator. The working group members will be informed before the printing order is given.

1.2 Purpose

The guideline serves all professional groups mentioned above who are directly or indirectly involved in the supply, care, nursing, and therapy of dialysis patients as well as the assessment of hygienic treatment standards.

Advantages for the User

The guideline provides a bridge between external documents (e.g. laws, guidelines, and regulations) and internal documents (e.g. hygiene plan). Processes which are embedded in quality management become clear. The guideline shall represent a reference book which links hygiene with quality management and gives answers to practical questions.

Advantages for the responsible organisation

Streamlining and optimising the process, prevention of mistakes and their resulting costs as well as the improvement of treatment safety are striven for. The areas of responsibility become clearer. Documented processes ease the tractability as well as the assessment and education of new employees. Analyses of weak points ensure increased treatment safety. The documented evidence of achieved treatment and quality results will become even more important in the future.

1.3 Usage and Assessment

1.3.1 Language of the Guideline

In this guideline, the modal auxiliary verb

- "must" (also "is/are to" or "has/have to") means that the observance of a requirement or the passing of an examination is an unconditional commandment (urgent recommendation which is scientifically proven: evidence-based) to observe these rules.
- "shall" means that the observance of a requirement or the passing of an examination is being recommended (recommenda-

tion according to expert opinion), however the compliance to these regulations is not an unconditional rule.
- "can/may/might" means that the observance of a requirement or the passing of an examination represents a possibility or an attempt at a solution.

In this form, the guideline linguistically follows other directives or norms closely.

Remark:
The Robert Koch Institute adds one more category IV in their Guidelines. These are based on laws and decrees[6].

1.3.2 State of Technology

The state of technology is referred to in Directive 93/42 EEC Medical Device Directive (MDD)[7]. "The state of technology is the stage of development of progressive processes, installations and operational modes which according to the prevailing opinion of leading specialists assures the attainment of the legally fixed goals. The codification of the state of technology also conforms to the regulations in other legal sectors (e.g. for machines which need Surveillance and X-ray installations) as well as the purpose of the present law in the interest of preventive health care. Thus it is also in accord with Council Directive 93/42/EEC. Likewise reference ismade there in Annex I to the state of the technology as it is generally recognised in EU countries."[8]

Remark:
The introduction of medical devices is regulated in Article 2 of the Medical Device Directive (MDD) [93/42/EEC] placing on the market and putting into service for all EU member states. This EC-Directive was put into national law by the

[6] Vorwort und Einleitung zur der Richtlinie für Krankenhaushygiene und Infektionsprävention. Bundesgesundheitsbl – Gesundheitsforsch – Gesundheitsschutz, 2004 (47): 409-411 (www.rki.de)

[7] Council Directive 93/42/EEC of 14th June 1993 on medical devices.

[8] Stellungnahme des Bundesrates zu § 17 Abs. 1 Nr. 6 des Entwurfes des Medizinproduktegesetzes. Bundestag-Drucksache 12/6991, 8. März 1994 (www.parlamentsspiegel.de)

Medical Devices Act (MPG). In § 14 (MPG) installation, operation, use and maintenance of medical devices is referred to § 37 paragraph 5 which authorises the Federal Ministry of Health to determine the installation, operation, use and maintenance of medical devices. This authorisation was realised through the Medical Device Operator Ordinance (MPBetreibV). The introduction is regulated in § 5 section 1 clause 2 and annex 1.

1.3.3 Approved Disinfectants and Procedures

If disinfectants and procedures are named, they refer to disinfectants and procedures which have been tested according to the present state of science and have been found effective; at least the limited spectrum of virucidal activity must have been proven. Sources for disinfectants are the lists of professional organisations, e.g. DGHM[9], RKI with the list for epidemic cases.[10]

Editorial note:
According to a joint statement of the Robert Koch Institute (RKI), the German Society for Hygiene and Microbiology (DGHM), the German Association against Virus Diseases (DVV) and the German Society of Hygiene and Microbiology, there is a distinction between a virucidal and a limited virucidal activity. The term "limited virucidal" describes the activity against enveloped viruses e.g. HBV, HCV, HIV, while "virucidal" has an additional activity against non-enveloped viruses e.g. polio viruses, HAV, Norwalk-like viruses[11].

[9] List certified according to the Directive for the examination of chemical disinfectants and accepted by the German Society for Hygiene and Microbiology (DGHM) to be effective disinfection procedures and procedures for the hygienic washing of hands. (www.dghm.de)

[10] List of the examined and accepted disinfectants and procedures by the Robert Koch Institute. Federal Health Gazette – Health Research – Health Protection, 2003 (46): 72-95. (www.rki.de)

[11] Examination and declaration of the effectiveness of disinfectants against viruses, statement of the Working Group Virucides of the Robert Koch Institute as well as the Committee of Experts "Virus Disinfection" of the German Association against Virus Diseases (DVV) and the Disinfectant Commission of the German Society for Hygiene and Microbiology (DGHM). Federal Health Gazette – Health Research – Health Protection, 2004 (47): 62-66 (www.rki.de)

1.4 Quality and Hygiene

1.4.1 Quality and Hygiene Management

Quality management has its origins in the manufacturing industry. It was there that ideas dealing with quality management were systematically developed and out of this a doctrine was developed which brought an enormous increase in quality for many companies.

The secret of its success lies in the fact that attention is not only directed to the quality of a product or the outcome of a service (outcome quality), but the quality desired is already systematically "planned in" and monitored during the development of a product or service. Furthermore, the general conditions and processes have to be attuned to the desired quality.

These findings can be directly applied to the hygiene management. Defined hygienic conditions can only be achieved when the required structural preconditions are fulfilled and all activities,

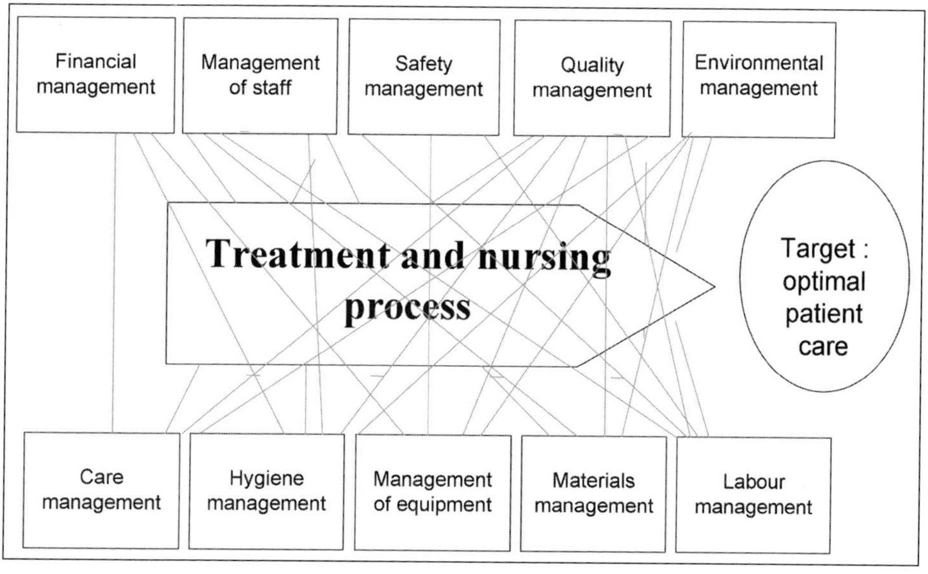

Fig. 1: Interconnectedness of different processes of a dialysis unit

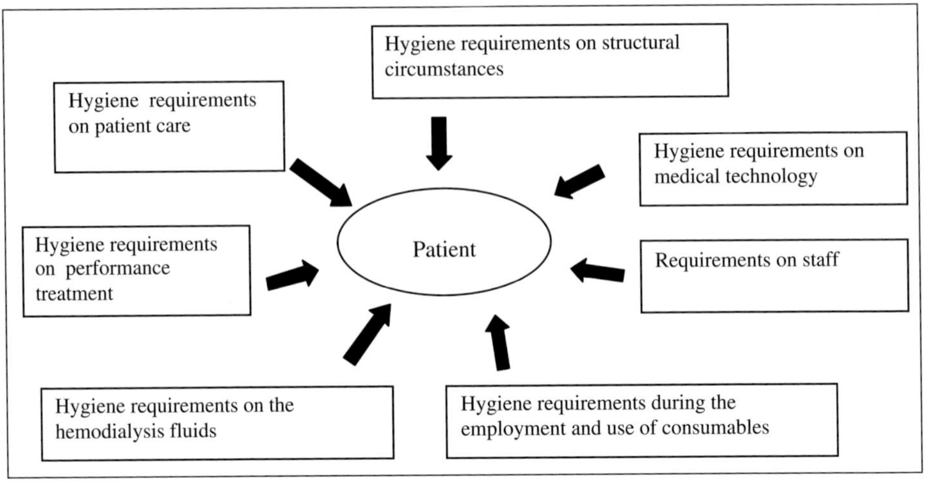

Fig. 2: Hygiene requirements and patient orientation

operations and processes are co-ordinated according to the results to be achieved. Among these are also processes which are not directly linked to hygiene or have apparently nothing to do with it. Therefore hygiene management shall always be seen as part of the whole management system, because many measures are mutually dependent and influence each other.

1.4.2 The Patient at the Centre of Attention

All processes and activities have to be in line with the expectations and requirements of the patient. It is thus logical that hygiene management also has to be focussed on the patient.

1.4.3 Continuous Quality Improvement of Hygiene in Dialysis

The basic principle of every functional management process is the continuous monitoring, further development and improvement of applied activities, procedures or actions. The system will then be adapted not only to constantly changing external conditions like new technologies or legal directives but also to internal changes.

Therefore hygiene management shall be set up according to the same principles. Regular monitoring for suitability and efficacy is indispensable.

This has been tried and tested in practice using the Deming or PDCA cycle; "plan, do, check, act"[12]. It obliges the user to regularly check the system for weak points and possible improvements.

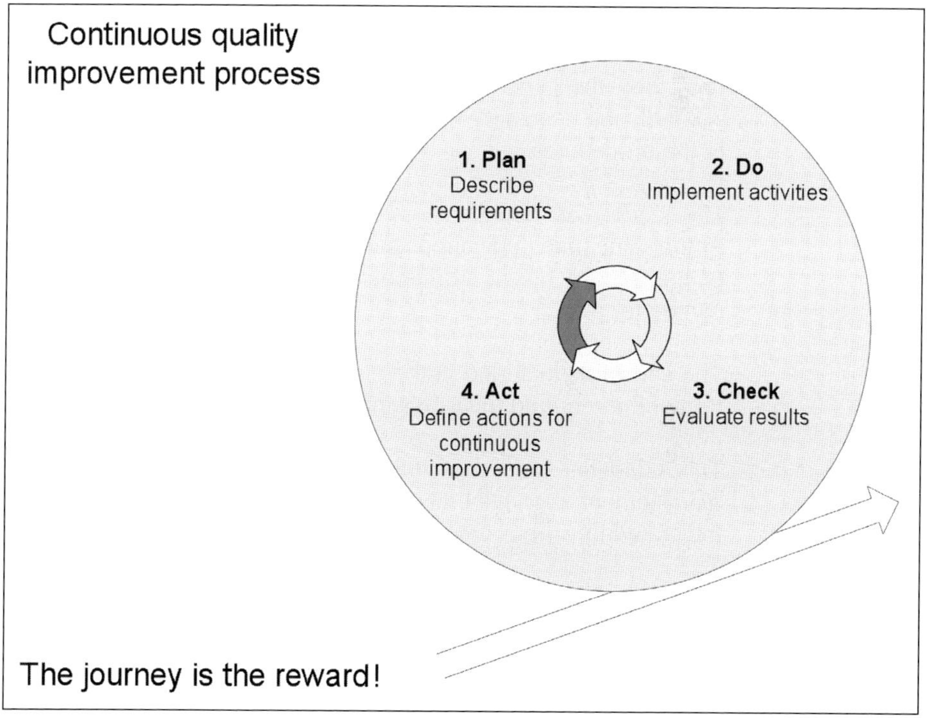

Fig. 3: The continuous improvement process

[12] www.qm-infocenter.de

The guideline supports the use of a continuous quality improvement process according to the PDCA principle:

- Description of the requirements
- Implementation activities
- Possibilities of evaluation of results
- Possible actions to be undertaken when nonconformity was observed.

1.4.4 Integration of the Guideline in a QM System

Hygiene measures are part of very different processes. If a hygiene management system is to be implemented in a dialysis unit, then the general processes have to be described first and secondly the necessary hygiene requirements are to be integrated in the procedures.

The reader can choose the relevant actions from the guideline. At the same time, indications are given how to evaluate the results of the actions taken. Additional suggestions for documentation can be used.

The checklists included in the guideline support the implementation of the required measures into practice.

This Guideline does not follow a particular model for quality management e.g. DIN EN ISO 9001:2000 so that it can be integrated in various QM systems.

Example of Integration for the Compendium to perform in the Process of Hemodialysis

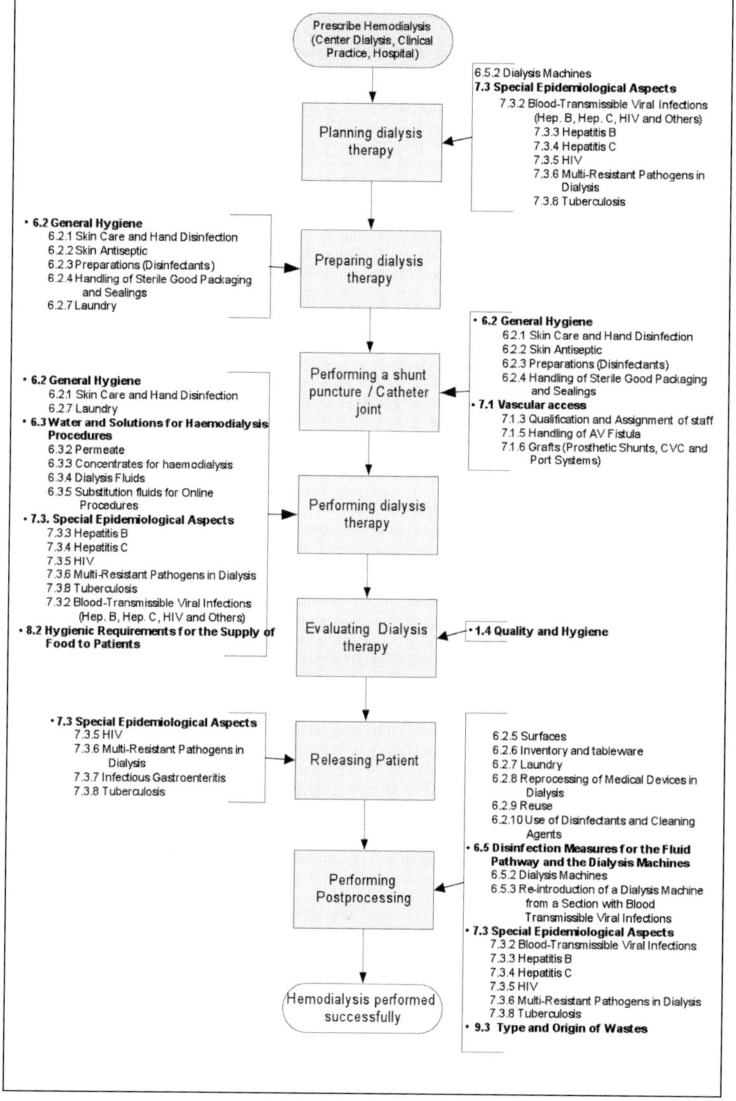

2 Legal Basis

2.1 Definition of Responsibilities

The responsible organisation bears the overall responsibility for the dialysis units operated. An appropriate organisational framework must be provided, which ensures a functioning work process, considering all relevant legal regulations for the organisation

- §§ 618 und 823 Bürgerliches Gesetzbuch – BGB (German Civil Code)
- § 62 Handelsgesetzbuch – HGB (Commercial Code)
- § 120 Gewerbeordnung – GewO (Industrial Code)
- §§ 9 and 130 Ordnungswidrigkeitengesetz – OwiG (Administrative Offences Act)
- §§ 13 and 14 Strafgesetzbuch – StGB (Penal Code)
- §§ 1, 8, 34, 35, 36, 42 and 43 Infektionsschutzgesetz – IfSG (Infections Protection Act)
- §§ 1, 2, and 4 Medizinproduktgesetz – MPG (Medical Devices Act)
- §§ 1-9 Medizinprodukt-Betreiberverordnung – MPBetreibV (Medical Device Operator Ordinance)
- §§ 3, 5-6 Arbeitsschutzgesetz – ArbSchG (Health & Safety at Work Law)
- §§ 2-14 Berufsgenossenschaftliche Vorschriften (BGV), Allgemeine Vorschriften – BGV A 1, Unfallverhütungsvorschrift, Grundsätze der Prävention (Regulations of the Employers' Liability Insurance Association)
- §§ 1-5, 7-16 Biostoffverordnung (Biological Agents Ordinance)
- Technische Regeln biologische Arbeitsstoffe ("Technical regulations for biological agents") (BGR 250/TRBA 250 „Biologische Arbeitsstoffe im Gesundheitswesen und in der Wohlfahrtspflege") ("Biological agents in the health care system and welfare work")
- TRBA 400 „Handlungsanleitung zur Gefährdungsbeurteilung bei Tätigkeiten mit biologischen Arbeitsstoffen" ("Operational instructions for risk assessment when handling biological agents")

- Richtlinien des Robert-Koch-Institutes (RKI-Richtlinien) (Directives of the Robert Koch Institute)
- Sterilgutversorgung DIN 58953-8 (Supply of sterile goods)

The responsible organisation must establish an appropriate organisational structure.

The following applies irrespective of any regulations of the duties and responsibility of the employer:
- Every individual is responsible for all her/his actions and what he/she decisively influences or can influence.
- The respective supervisors act on behalf of the employer and within their field of responsibility.

2.2 Responsible Organisation

The "responsible organisation" can be a legal entity, e.g. diocese, association, foundation, society as well as natural persons, e.g. group practise of physicians or a physician in private practise.

2.3 Equality of Occupational Health and Patient Safety

Responsibility in the sense of "responsible organisation" involves the implementation of the existing hygiene requirements for patients and staff safety.

All those concerned in provision of dialysis care are responsible for their safety and health at work and shall act according to the instructions and directives of the employer. Staff members also have to take care of the safety and health of patients and others involved. It is within this framework that the machines, tools, working materials, means of conveyance and other materials as well as safety devices and personal protective equipment placed at their disposal are to be used according to the regulations[13].

2.4 Biological Agents Ordinance (BioStoffV)

2.4.1 The Biological Agents Ordinance and its Effects on the Operation of a Dialysis Centre

The BioStoffV concerning safety and health protection when working with biological agents was issued as an ordinance to the Health & Safety at Work Law and it is the implementation of a European Directive (90/679/EWG) into German law. It applies to all sectors in which employees handle biological agents.

In terms of this ordinance, biological agents are bacteria and similar organisms, viruses, parasites and fungi.

Blood and other body fluids are actually no biological agents. They are regarded as human material which can still be contaminated with biological agents. The exact definition of biological agents can be found in § 2 of the BioStoffV. They are listed in the joint classification (Annex III of Directive 2000/54 of the European Parliament and Council of 18th September 2000[14]) while taking into consideration their potential danger. Also specific circumstances are described in the technical regulations for biological agents (TRBA).

The Biological Agents Ordinance differentiates between specific and non-specific handling of biological agents.

Remark:
Only the non-specific handling of biological working materials is relevant in the public health service sector and thus for dialysis. It is for this reason that here too, only the above will be dealt with.

---

[13] vergl. § 15 Abs. 1 und 2 Arbeitsschutzgesetz – ArbSchG, http://bundesrecht.juris.de sowie Medizinproduktegesetz – MPG mit seinen Verordnungen.

[14] http://europa.eu.int/eur-lex

2.4.2 Risk Groups

According to § 3 of the BioStoffV, biological agents are divided into four risk groups based on their corresponding risks of infection:

- Risk group 1: Biological agents which are unlikely to cause human disease
- Risk group 2: Biological agents which can cause human disease and might be a hazard to workers; spreading of the agent into the community is unlikely; usually effective prophylaxis or treatment is available
- Risk group 3: Biological agents which can cause severe human disease and present a serious hazard to workers; there may be a risk of spreading to the community, but usually effective prophylaxis or treatment is available
- Risk group 4: Biological agents which can cause severe human disease and pose a serious hazard to workers; there may be a high risk of spreading to the community; there is usually no effective prophylaxis or treatment available.

2.4.3 Risk Assessment

The BiostoffV obliges the employer to carry out risk assessment in the working areas where biological materials are relevant. In this case the TRBA 400[15] classification "Operational instructions for risk assessment when handling biological agents" have to be applied. Substantial procedural guidelines regarding the assessment of activities, classification of risk groups, the classification of protection levels and the necessary protective measures and also for many other questions are found in the BGR 250/TRBA 250 "Biological agents in the health care system and welfare work."

[15] www.baua.de (Bundesanstalt für Arbeitsschutz und Arbeitsmedizin – BAuA)

2.4.4 Operating Instructions and Instruction of Employees

Working area and subject-related operating instructions are to be based on the risk assessment instructions for specific work areas and have to be agent-specific and the employees have to be instructed accordingly.

2.4.5 Notification of the Supervisory Body

A notification of the responsible supervisory body and the obligation to register also covers non-specific handling when the conditions stated in § 13 section 5 are fulfilled. However, such a case will be an exception in a dialysis centre.

2.4.6 Occupational Health Surveillance and Immunisation

The employer has to ensure that employees working with biological agents undergo occupational health surveillance before starting work and afterwards at regular intervals. These examinations are compulsory when the job is listed in annex IV of the BiostoffV. As a result it implies that at least testing for HBV and HCV biological agents is to be done. The occupational health surveillance check-up is to be carried out by an authorised physician in compliance with the professional trade association principle for occupational health examinations, chapter G-42 "Infectious diseases". The employee is to be offered vaccination if an effective vaccine is available[16]. Obliging the employee to take the vaccination cannot be derived from the BioStoffV [17, 18].

[16] BGR 250/TRBA 250: Biologische Arbeitsstoffe im Gesundheitswesen und in der Wohlfahrtspflege, (www.bgw-online.de)

[17] BioStoffV § 20 Abs. 3

[18] IfSG (Infections Protection Act) § 15a

2.5 The Hygiene Plan

2.5.1 Legal Aspects

The instructions of the employer for patient and staff safety are to be defined in writing in the hygiene plan[19]. The employees are to be instructed about its content at regular intervals.[20]

The established rules of hygiene and occupational health and safety especially the guidelines of the RKI, the Infections Protection Act (IfSG), the BioStoffV as well as the drawing-up of a risk analysis of all the work sections must be respected when drafting and setting the content:

- Infektionsschutzgesetz – IfSG (Infections Protection Act)
- Lebensmittel- und Bedarfsgegenständegesetz – LMBG (Foodstuffs and Consumer Goods Law)
- Lebensmittelhygieneverordnung – LMHV (Foodstuff Hygiene Ordinance)
- Gefahrstoffverordnung – GefstoffV (Ordinance on Hazardous Substances)
- Arzneimittelgesetz – AMG (German Pharmaceutical Act)
- Europäische Pharmakopoe – Europharm (European Pharmacopoeia)
- Trinkwasserverordnung – TrinkwV (Drinking Water Ordinance)
- Chemikaliengesetz – ChemG (Chemicals Act)
- Technische Regeln für biologische Arbeitsstoffe – TRBA (Technical Regulations for Biological Agents)
- Kreislaufwirtschaft- und Abfallgesetz mit seinen Verordnungen – KrW-/AbfG (Waste and Recycling Act with its bylaws)

[19] IfSG (Infections Protection Act) § 36; BGR 250/TRBA 250, ch. 4.1.2.3
[20] BioStoffV (Biological Agents Ordinance) § 12; BGR 250/TRBA 250, ch. 5.2

2.5.2 Case Sample of a Hygiene Plan[21]

A hygiene plan shall for example contain the following components:

2.5.2.1 General Information about the Dialysis Unit

- Name(s) and address of the operator
- Naming the nurse manager and the infection control specialist, the safety officer and the occupational health specialist (depending on the type of unit/hospital and organisation)
- Dates for regular revisions
- Documentation file for annual staff instruction and signature record

2.5.2.2 Occupational Safety and Health

The implementation of the Biological Agents Ordinance (determining the type of job, the risk group, the safety level) has to take place for employees and external persons:
- Occupational health check-up with instructions concerning occupational safety and health
- Occupational health check-up and deadlines for follow-ups
- Immunisation
- Accident reporting, e.g. minor accidents, occupational accidents, occupational diseases, procedure in case of needlestick injuries and possible post-exposure prophylaxis (PEP)
- Skin care and protection plan

2.5.2.3 Organisational and Function-Specific Instructions for the Prevention of Infections

- Hand hygiene, e.g. ban wearing jewellery, short unpainted fingernails, cleanliness
- Isolation or quarantine regulations

[21] IfSG (Infections Protection Act)

- Measures for puncturing of shunts and grafts, insertion and connection of catheters, e.g. requirements on the working environment, protective clothing
- Aseptic measures for changing the dressing of catheter exits, drainage bag (PD), or transitional system (PD)
- Regular checking for HBV, HCV and HIV infections including schedule and parameters
- Documentation and incidence report system according to §§ 6 and 8 of the Infections Protection Act (IfSG)

2.5.2.4 Organisation of Cleaning and Disinfection

- Hand disinfection – importance, when, what with, how
  Editorial note: European Standard DIN EN 1499 defines "handwashing", EN 1500 edition 1997 defines "hand disinfection"
- Skin disinfection – importance, when, what with, how
- Surface cleaning and disinfection – importance, what, when, what with, how
- Laundering and disinfection of the linen, including hygiene certificate of the laundry

2.5.2.5 Reprocessing of Medical Devices

- Risk assessment and classification of the medical devices to be reprocessed defining the responsibilities for all steps undertaken in the reprocessing

2.5.2.6 Monitoring and Measures Safeguarding the Microbiological Quality of Drinking Water and Dialysis Fluids

- Permeate (or dialysis or product water): Definition of quality requirements, sampling frequency, sites, procedures and transport, the laboratory commissioned to do the examinations and

actions to be undertaken in case of non-conformity of quality standards
- Dialysis concentrate from central distribution system: requirements as for permeate
- Drinking water: requirements according to the Drinking Water Ordinance (TrinkwV)

2.5.2.7 Food Hygiene

- Instructions according to § 43 section 1 and 4 of the Infection Protection Act with documentation
- Personal hygiene, e.g. wearing of protective clothing, hand hygiene
- Separation of clean and unclean work areas
- Storage facility with monitoring and documentation of temperature and expiry dates
- Forbidden to store foodstuffs, chemicals (cleaning agents and disinfectants) and medications in the same place
- Cleaning and disinfection of working materials, devices and surfaces

2.5.2.8 Waste Disposal

For each of the occurring waste types the following criteria have to be described:
- specific characteristics, the safety measures to be observed by the staff, the collection bins, the transport within the facility, the collecting points, the pick-up rhythm and the waste disposal company in charge:
- Wastes which can be recycled after utilisation e.g. films, cartons, empty cans,
- Non-infectious wastes which are not allowed to be recycled (no sharps)
- Non-infectious but injury-causing dangerous wastes ("sharps")
- Infectious wastes with a description of type and origin
- Left over food

2.5.2.9 Action in Case of Accidents and Incidents

Appropriate materials and equipment for notification has to be provided for the case of accidents of patients and staff. Instructions for correct use must be given.

The hygiene plan shall contain adequate indications of e.g.:
- Emergency telephone as well as other devices for notification of emergencies
- First Aid facilities and competent persons
- Internal as well as external rescue centres
- In-house system of accident reporting
- Documentation and registration forms
- Incident reporting system according to the Medical Device Operator Ordinance (MPBetreibV), reaction to transfusions, undesired action of drugs and complications arising from vaccinations.
- etc.

2.5.3 Appendix/Notice

- Disinfection plans for the various sections e.g. treatment, kitchen, technicians work room, laboratory, disposal
- Waste disposal plans for the various sections e.g. treatment, kitchen, technique, laboratory, disposal
- Skin care and protection plan
- Various operating instructions for dealing with dangerous preparations and dangerous substances e.g. disinfectants
- Instruction leaflet on needlestick injuries
- Instruction leaflet on post-exposure prophylaxis

3 Structural Requirements

3.1 Goal and Rationale

The goal of defining the structural requirements when planning new facilities is to avoid structural mistakes which can have an effect on hygiene and possible resulting costs.

3.2 Space Required

The following space/partition is recommended for every dialysis unit:

3.2.1 Physician's Rooms

The rooms shall be located near the treatment areas.

3.2.2 Treatment Sections

There shall be a distinction between infectious and non-infectious treatment sections[22].

Remark:
Patients with the following infections may need separate treatment rooms: HBV, HCV, MRE, HIV, tuberculosis, etc.

[22] Anlagen zur Richtlinie für Krankenhaushygiene und Infektionsprävention (www.rki.de)

3.2.3 Haemodialysis (HD) Treatment Section with hygienically clean work station

- Treatment room
  The space required for each dialysis place must be calculated in such a way that every treatment place can be reached unhindered from three sides. Due to special needs for medical/technical equipment, a sufficient distance of 1.30 m between the beds or dialysis chairs must be planned. Transporting patients with a trolley must be possible.

Other rooms are:
- Patients' monitoring room/office or staff office
- Multipurpose emergency treatment room with connections for HD/PD devices
- General workroom
- Rooms for wet work activities, one of those shall be reserved for infectious patients
- Examination room in case others in the immediate vicinity cannot be used
- Room with emergency diagnostic equipment if necessary
- Room for the preparation and distribution of food

3.2.4 Treatment Section for Intermittent Peritoneal Dialysis (IPD)

- Staff office
- Multipurpose emergency treatment room with connections for HD/PD devices
- General workroom
- Rooms for wet work activities, one of those shall be reserved for infectious patients
- Examination room in case others in the immediate vicinity cannot be used
- Room with emergency diagnostic equipment if necessary

3.2.5 HD-/PD-Training

- Training and treatment room
- "Wet room" or a room to drain used PD, HF or HD fluid insofar as a corresponding room cannot be jointly used in the general section for treatment
- Office

3.2.6 Open Rooms for Patients

- Waiting area/lounge
- Patients' wardrobe and changing rooms separated according to sex
- Toilets, one of which shall be for infectious patients if necessary
- WC adapted to the needs of disabled persons

3.2.7 Open Rooms for Staff

They must be furnished in accordance with the Industrial Safety Act, Workplace Ordinance and the Accident Prevention Regulations, especially the BGR 250/TRBA 250.

3.2.8 Dialysis for Children

Additional space is required in dialysis units for children.

3.2.9 Technical Services Room:

- Water processing room
- Room for central concentrate supply if necessary

- Room for maintenance of devices with connections for HD and PD devices if necessary
- Electrical engineering room
- Room for an emergency generator if necessary

3.2.10 Administration

Administrative rooms depending on the needs

3.2.11 General Utility Management

The structural measures for guaranteeing the general housing technology supply and disposal (electricity, heating, gas, water, waste) are orientated towards whether and how the facility for the treatment of dialysis can be incorporated into the existing infrastructures of a house. The existing building laws and constructional norms are to be observed in all the new housing technological facilities to be constructed.

3.2.12 Supply and Disposal Rooms

- Storerooms (number and size depending on the supply system)
- Distribution kitchen with storeroom if necessary
- Storage space for devices and beds outside of the areas used for general treatment and circulation
- Dirty linen room
- Waste collection points/areas according to the waste disposal system
- Room for e.g. bed-pan cleaning and disinfecting machines if not installed in another suitable place
- Room for cleaning utensils

3.3 Room Set-up and Installations

Wall surfaces and floors of rooms used medically have to be smooth, watertight, and washable. Disinfection with disinfectants and disinfection procedures must be possible[23]; in case of plagues, also with disinfection procedures which are recognised by the RKI. In addition, floors and wall connections are supposed to be made waterproof. Floor covering shall be anti-static.

Sufficient wash hand basins and dispensers for disinfectants must be available in the treatment rooms.

Rooms for the water supply facility and the concentrate supply are rooms for medical utilisation. The structural execution as well as the cleaning and maintenance must be done in accordance with their special hygienic status.

The dialysis-specific installations must be carried out after special consideration of the hygienic requirements. Permeate and sewage pipes shall be easily accessible, e.g. for the possibility of inspections. Other pipes are to be concealed or lead into closed canals whose external walls can be disinfected[24]. Heaters and air passages shall be installed in a way that they can be easily cleaned and disinfected.

3.4 Sanitary Facilities

Water fittings which can be used without using the hands have to be installed in places for washing hands. The jet of water shall not lead directly into the siphon[25]. This does not apply to domestic sections.

[23] Anlage zur Richtlinie für Krankenhaushygiene und Infektionsprävention (www.rki.de) BGR 250/TRBA 250, ch. 4.1.1.3 and ch. 4.2.2

[24] DIN EN 793, VDE (Association for Electrical, Electronic & Information Technologies) 0750 Part 211- NEW: DIN EN ISO 11197 from mid 05

[25] Anlagen zur Richtlinie für Krankenhaushygiene und Infektionsprävention (www.rki.de)

3.5 Requirements on the Indoor Air

If technical indoor air equipment (RLT) is needed, the constructional regulations in accordance with DIN 1946-4[26] are to be respected.

Separate appliances like ventilators, fan heaters, cooling units and indoor air humidifiers are not technical indoor air equipment within the context of this regulation.

These appliances have to be operated in a way that no microorganisms can accumulate inside and that they cannot spread any chemicals into the ambient air. The microbiological composition of the indoor air within the treatment unit is not supposed to disadvantageously change through the use of such appliances.

3.6 Sewage System

During the installation of the sewage pipes leading through the dialysis unit the danger of an obstruction or blockage in the flow of fluids must be avoided.

The following shall be taken into account during the installation of pipes:

- Diameter of pipes
- Angle of inclination
- Corrosion-resistant materials
- Inspection access

Remark:
A too small angle of inclination of the sewage pipes and the resultant reduction in the speed of flow facilitates sedimentation in the drainage system of the dialysis. Practical experience has shown that if these conditions are not met, "obstructions" will always occur in the sewage pipes leading to a reflux of contaminated dialysate right back into the dialysis unit. If cast iron pipes are used, it is advisable

[26] www.bauregeln.de

to regularly carry out visual inspections to check for signs of corrosion as far as possible and if necessary to do maintenance work on the damaged parts at the right time. HD-PE pipes for example shall be used when installing new sewage pipes.

Drainage sinks are to be cleaned using certified surface disinfectants and procedures.

Domestic sewage pipes do not need any disinfection.

4 Medical and Technological Requirements in Haemodialysis

4.1 Goal and Rationale

Quality of life of dialysis patients is not only influenced by medical and nursing care but also by the quality of technical equipment[27]. Short and long term complications in patients can occur as a result of hygienic weaknesses in the medical equipment and their installations. These complications have to be avoided[28].

A high degree of functionality and user-friendliness of the medical equipment shall be guaranteed.

4.2 Water Purification

The operator is responsible for maintenance and operation of the entire system. The guidelines laid down in the Medical Products Act (MPG) and its regulations are to be respected. This applies especially for systems with individual components from different manufacturers. The product information concerning compatibility with other medical devices has to be considered.

Remark:
According to EN 60601, the operator becomes the manufacturer when he combines different medical devices.

[27] Baz, M. et al.: Using ultrapure water in haemodialysis delays carpal tunnel syndrome. Artificial Organs, 1991 (14 (11)): 681-685

[28] Nystrand, R.: Contamination of the fluid systems and the life of microbes. EDTNA/ERCA Journal XXVII, July-September 2001 (3): 145-151

4.2.1 General Requirements

In general the following shall be taken into consideration:

- Safe and verified procedures for disinfection of reverse osmosis and distribution system with safe and easy to handle methods
- Heat-disinfectable, automatic water purification and supply systems when new systems are to be installed
- Materials, connection technique and pipe installation without or with minimal dead space design.

4.2.2 Requirements on Installation and Planning

With the transition from urban or communal drinking water network into the domestic installation, responsibility for the water quality is passed to the provider[29].

Depending on the results of the analysis of drinking water and considering the expected water quality, the manufacturer of the reverse osmosis unit has to define the requirements for the pre-treatment.
Pre-treatment components which can contain particle filters, softener, activated charcoal filter, sand bed filter and/or iron reducer serve to protect the reverse osmosis membrane.
Regular disinfection of pre-treatment units is not necessary.
Maintenance of the microbiological quality of the permeate after the reverse osmosis membrane is of utmost concern.
The quality of the required permeate (see ch. 11.3) determines the necessary measures. These measures are influenced by local environmental variables like temperature, pressure/flow, capacity, and the analysis of drinking water.
A separation of the pipework, e.g. "free outlet" (air gap) or pipe separator, must be installed within central water purification units.

[29] Verordnung zur Novellierung der Trinkwasserverordnung vom 21. Mai 2001. BGB I Nr. 24 vom 28. Mai 2001

The manufacturer has to provide evidence that every single medical device is installed in accordance with the legal requirements and that it delivers the specified quality. If a combination of medical devices is installed by the manufacturer, the manufacturer has to provide all information on how the whole system can be handled in view of maintaining the hygienic quality[30].

Remark:
No supplier of a medical device system will guarantee the faultless function to the provider if the system contains elements from another source (manufacturer) than his own. The supplier defines the requirements for the "company in combination with other medical devices" in his instructions for use and thereby forwards the definition of the interface to the operator. The operator bears the responsibility for the maintenance and operation when there is a combination of medical devices from different suppliers. If all the connected medical devices come from one single supplier, the buyer or organisation can request that the supplier provides a description on how to maintain the hygienic quality for the complete system provided by him.

4.2.3 Reverse Osmosis

The microbiological quality of permeate is defined by the technical layout of the system as well as by the regular quality assurance measures.

4.2.4 Single Patient Reverse Osmosis

At present, there is no consistent procedure for hygienic maintenance of Single Patient Water Treatment Unit or Reverse Osmosis devices especially in intermittent home dialysis application. Regular preventive monthly disinfection is recommended. Chemical disinfection is the current standard to disinfect these systems. Automatic heat-disinfecting systems shall be the standard in the future.

---

[30] Directive 93/42/EEC of the Council of 14th June 1993 on Medical Devices (www.bfarm.de)

Editorial Remark: Increased frequency of preventive disinfection might be necessary if microbiological results are out of specification

4.2.5 Supply Units and Connection Systems

The integration of the permeate inlet tube to the dialysis machine into the disinfection cycle is possible in modern systems and shall be realised in new installations. Heat-disinfection procedures are the preferred procedures. The connected dialysis machines shall have cleansing and disinfection programmes which allow procedures that can incorporate these two elements in a "central disinfection" system.

In case the inlet tube connector is disconnected from the permeate piping system, the dry connector on the media panel circuit (wall) and the dry connector of the supply tube have to be thoroughly disinfected, i.e. sprayed or wiped off with a disinfectant and dried as much as possible. The exposure time of the disinfectant has to be respected.

Remark:
Present connection systems for permeate inflow and drain, the so-called "free dialysate outlet flow" (air gap) are mostly fitted close to each other for reasons of practicability. During the planning and construction of the inflow and drain units supplier and provider shall consider the prevention of contamination of permeate and central concentrate connectors through the fluid spills from the drain air gap ("free dialysate outflow").

4.3 Dialysis Machines

4.3.1 General

The back-flow as a re-contamination from the machine into the permeate circuit pipe has to be prevented through suitable means by the manufacturer[31] of the dialysis machines. The dialysate outflow tube has to be connected to the room drain piping system using an air gap of at least 20 mm[32].

4.3.2 Surfaces

External materials have to be resistant to surface disinfectants. Surfaces have to be easy to clean and disinfect, non-accessible spaces and gaps shall be avoided by design as far as possible. Critical parts such as dialyser couplings and concentrate connectors shall also be integrated into the cleaning/disinfection process[33] in a suitable way.

4.3.3 Hydraulic Circuit

Due to the chemical reactions of the concentrate components, the retention time of ready-mixed dialysis fluid in the hydraulic circuit has to be kept as short as possible. Therefore the total volume of the hydraulic circuit is to be designed as small as possible through minimal diameters and short tube connections. For hygienic reasons and for optimal rinsing and flushing of disinfectants, there must not be any dead spaces.

The materials have to comply with the DIN EN ISO 10993-1 (biological assessment of medical devices). The conduit of the dialysis fluid shall be designed in a way that no dialysate can mix with

---

[31] EN 1717:2000 Protection of drinking water from contamination in drinking water installations and general requirements to safety installations for dealing with the prevention of drinking water from contamination through backflow; DIN VDE 0753-4 Instructions for use of dialysis units, presently being revised

[32] EN 1717:2000 Protection of drinking water from contamination in drinking water installations and general requirements to safety installations for dealing with the prevention of drinking water from drinking water contamination through backflow; DIN VDE 0753-4 Instructions for use of dialysis units, presently being revised

[33] VDE 0750 Teil 2-16: Medizinische elektrische Geräte: Besondere Festlegungen an Hämodialyse-, Hämodiafiltrations- und Hämofiltrationsgeräte

the fresh dialysis fluid. This is the meaning of a so called "single pass machine".

The disinfection of the hydraulic circuit of a dialysis machine has to integrate all components that have contact with fluids. All materials have to be resistant to the recommended disinfectants and cleaning products available and the disinfection procedures specified by the manufacturer. In case critical elements, i.e. air separators, filters or other, need to be part of the design, then these must be disinfected and safely rinsed as part of the disinfection/ cleaning process.

Dialysis machines have to indicate to the user if the disinfection process was disturbed or interrupted as well as if the process did not take place at all. An indication of the last complete disinfection shall be indicated by the machine.

The user shall not be able to change or override the fixed concentration of use, time of disinfection, time of rinsing (compulsory rinsing), but the procedure shall be revisable.

Mandatory rinsing has to take place depending on the potential risk of the disinfection or cleaning procedure.

If the machine is equipped with a separate operating mode "cleaning", the cleaning process shall not work in a "recirculation" mode because dissolved or dispatched particles of deposits downstream could be spread across the hydraulic system. In order to achieve optimal effectiveness with the used agent, a pre-selected temperature of for example 80 °C hot/37 °C warm is advisable in the cleaning process. After a isolated cleaning process the hydraulic system of the dialysis machine must be disinfected. Disinfection procedures shall be programmed in a way that the use of electricity, water and chemicals is minimised without compromising the hygienic safety in critical areas.

Through such measures it can be ensured that every treatment takes place under the equal and comparable hygienic conditions.

4.3.4 Dialysis Machines – Inflow and Drain Connections

Interfaces to be used for permeate and concentrate transfers are the connections fixed on tubes to the machine. These connectors must be easy to handle and impossible to mix-up.
For hygienic reasons, there shall be suitable fittings on the machine for holding the disconnected supply pipes.
The permeate supply tubes shall be manufactured, stored and mounted under hygienic conditions. They shall be disinfected or changed at regular intervals.

Remark:
Regular disinfection/hot cleaning of the permeate supply tube is possible only in some elder or recently developed dialysis machines. The application and regular change of Ultrafilters in the dialysis fluid circuit can significantly reduce the risk of contaminating the dialysis membrane and the patients[34].

Direct connection of concentrate pickup tubes to the supply circuit through a standardised coupling and integrating this supply line into the disinfection cycle is recommended.

Remark:
An integration of the concentrate inlet tube into the disinfection procedure is only possible in newly developed dialysis machines and through additional installations. The application and regular change of Ultrafilters in the dialysis fluid circuit can significantly reduce the risk of contaminating the dialysis membrane and the patients.

Holders and connections for cartridges such as sodium hydrogen carbonate (sodium bicarbonate) powder have to be included into the disinfection cycle.
A hygienic weakness in some types of machines is the lack of integrating the concentrate pickup tubes into the disinfection cycle.
Each dialysis machine shall have its own drain outlet into the domestic sewage pipe system.

---

[34] European Best Practice Guidelines for Haemodialysis, Section IV: Dialysis fluid purity. VI. 3 Haemodialysis proportioning machine. Nephrol. Dial. Transplant, 2002 (17 (7)): 49-50 (http://ndt.oxfordjournals.org)

4.3.5 Sample Collection Ports

The manufacturer shall equip the dialysis machine with suitable sampling ports.

4.3.6 Accessories

Concentrate tubes of machines which do not integrate such tubes in the disinfection circuit have to be at least rinsed with permeate after being used and, if necessary cleaned and disinfected. After that, the concentrate tubes can be left to dry or can be preserved in a solution which suppresses the microbial growth i.e. the acid concentrate component. There must be enough pickup tubes available in order to guarantee an easy and safe handling.

Remark:
The pickup tubes for the bicarbonate concentrate are more prone to contamination because of the low osmolarity of the bicarbonate. All the suggested proposals mentioned till now, i.e. storage in acid concentrate, rinsing with permeate or chemical disinfection followed by rinsing with permeate and dry storage meet problems in the procedure. Their effectiveness is not documented to date.

4.3.7 Operating Manual

All relevant parameters related to the hygienic quality of the dialysis machine, such as the recommended disinfection procedures, disinfectants, dwell and rinsing times and handling are to be defined clearly in the operating manual[35]. Furthermore, reference shall be made to the validation of procedures or relevant expert reports.

A basic principle when developing new dialysis machines shall not only be sufficient effectiveness of disinfection procedures and safe treatments, but also minimal exposure to chemicals for staff, patients and environment.

[35] Directive 93/42/EEC of the Council from 14th June 1993 on Medical devices (www.bfarm.de)

5 Staff requirements

5.1 Goal and Rationale

Staff that have competent knowledge and skills ensure a high quality treatment for their patients. Staff must ensure that they carry out timely audit measures in order to avoid a reduction in quality. The employer/provider has to provide the framework for a structured and target-oriented transmission of knowledge[36].

Hygiene is an elementary component of quality assurance in dialysis treatment. Omission or failure can put patients and staff acutely at risk, but are in any case a threat to the patients' quality of life on a long-term basis. In-depth education, initial and repeated instruction and training are mandatory for all staff involved.

Mistakes reduce the treatment outcome and limit the optimal use of resources. For the patient mistakes may mean hospitalisation and deterioration of the prognosis. Education and training promote preventative thinking and acting, and build up the patient's confidence. Mistakes and ignorance provoke criticism, reduce the motivation, generate additional costs and waste resources.

5.2 Staffing Structure

There shall be a wide range of professional groups involved with the subject of hygiene and infection control in dialysis treatment. Besides the physicians and nursing staff who are directly involved in patient care, there are many other professional groups who are involved at various stages.

During the planning phase the range of professionals involved includes providers, authorities, architects, construction companies, equipment manufacturers dealing with companies respon-

[36] MPBetreibV § 2

sible for the sanitary facilities, such as water supply and water treatment. In the day to day operations, those involved primarily are the physician(s) in charge, nursing staff, medical and nursing assistants, technicians, and cleaning staff as well as hygienists, microbiologists, manufacturers and distributors of dialysis supply.

All persons and members of professional groups directly involved in the care and treatment of dialysis patients and who operate medical devices are supposed to have been instructed in activities of the haemodialysis field. They must have sufficient knowledge on hygienic and technical requirements as well as having knowledge of the problem areas in dialysis treatment[37].

5.3 Initial and Annual Instruction

The joint work of the multi-professional group on the "guideline" has proven that the level of knowledge on the subject of hygiene and dialysis show variations. Individual professional or specialist associations have established curricula and job descriptions in which references are made to the requirements for hygiene in dialysis.

The responsibility of management is to ensure initial and regular instructions and documentation, as well as evaluation of the results and implementation of correcting measures. The management must constantly keep up to date with the current state of knowledge.

The comprehensive and extensive instruction and professional education of staff who are directly responsible for patient care comprises different levels:

- Instruction on the dialysis machines and installations according to the Medical Devise Act (MPG)[38]

---

[37] MPBetreibV § 5; BioStoffV § 12; GefahrstoffV § 14; DIN VDE 0753-4 Anwendungsregeln für Hämodialysegeräte (presently being revised)

[38] MPG § 14 und § 37 Abs. 5 und MPBetreibV § 5 Abs. 1 Ziffer 2 und Anlage 1

- Instruction on the hygiene plan including the disinfection plans and the handling of hazardous substances, etc.[39]
- Continuous education based on a education concept in which all instructions are documented
- Theoretical education based on a curriculum for all who are involved in the direct treatment and care of patients.

Regular and repeated instruction in the field of hygiene and equipment technology is necessary in order to deepen, update and expand knowledge. Some of this instruction has to be done annually and some immediately when there are changes in practice.

The instruction of staff working in the dialysis unit has to take place immediately after the annual revision of the hygiene plan. A previous internal audit of the internal hygiene standards with the help of an audit sheet, facilitates the establishment of deviations and problems as well as the establishment of the content of the instructions and the discussion on necessary corrective measures.

Every instruction and education has to be documented with regards to the content and the participants.

[39] GefahrstoffV § 14; BGR 250/TRBA 250, ch. 5.2

Overview of Target Groups for Initial and Regular Instruction

Target Group	Instruction/Education	Initial and repeated Instruction
Dialysis staff • All nursing staff	Instructions • Hygiene plan • Medical Device Act Education concept[40, 41] Theoretical education	Annually and in case of changes
• Assistants	Instructions • Hygiene plan • Medical Product Act if necessary Education	Annually and in case of changes
Patients	Education concept Patients' hygiene	In case of changes
Cleaning companies • Cleaning workers	Basics, e.g. hygiene plan	In case of changes
Provider and assigned departments or service providers i.e. architects, planning department, logistic management, dialysis technicians	Knowledge of the hygiene plan, "guideline" and other literature	In case of changes
Equipment manufacturer • Dialysis technician • Development department	Knowledge of the hygiene plan, "guideline" and other literature	In case of changes
Staff member responsible for hygiene	Knowledge of the hygiene plan, guideline and other literature	In case of changes
Other service providers • Laboratories • Authorities • Occupational medical services	Knowledge of the legal regulations, "guideline" and other literature	In case of changes

[40] DKG = Deutsche Krankenhaus Gesellschaft: „Muster für eine landesrechtliche Ordnung der Weiterbildung und Prüfung zu Krankenschwestern, Krankenpflegern, Kinderkrankenschwestern und Kinderkrankenpflegern auf dem Gebiet der Nephrologie", das Krankenhaus 1995 (5): Redaktionsbeilage

[41] Curriculum Bundesärztekammer für Arzthelferinnen und Krankenschwestern in der Dialyse

6 Requirements for the Organisation

6.1 Goal and Rationale

The treatment process must be characterised by professional behaviour in view of the prevention of infections and suitable measures for the improvement of hygiene.

Following issues have direct influence on the quality of treatment as well as the long-term quality of life and life expectancy of patients[42].

6.2 General Hygiene

6.2.1 Skin Care and Hand Disinfection

6.2.1.2 Skin Care and Protection

Healthy skin is a precondition for effective hand hygiene. The protective measures to be undertaken when skin is at risk to be endangered as a result of working in moist milieu are laid down in the Technical Regulations for Hazardous Substances (TRGS)[43].

The measures apply to employees working in moist milieu with their hands for at least 2 hours per day. Suitable gloves are to be worn. Equipment for personal protection, cleaning agents, protective agents and care products have to be provided by the employer for the employees. Skin care plan has to be defined depending on the expected noxious substances. Based on the skin care plan

[42] Stenvinkel P. et al.: Strong association between malnutrition, inflammation, and atherosclerosis in chronic renal failure. Kidney Int. 1999 (55): 1899-1911

[43] TRGS 531: Gefährdung der Haut durch Arbeiten im feuchten Milieu (Feuchtarbeit)

a selection of products for cleaning, protection and skin care must be provided for use.

6.2.1.2 Hand Hygiene

Effective measures in the hygiene of hands is probably the most important measure in the prevention of infections. The respective guidelines of the RKI[44] have to be adhered to. Generally, a hygienic disinfection of the hands without previous washing is sufficient. Preconditions for effective hand hygiene are short fingernails trimmed to the finger tips with surfaces which are not cracked or polished.

Remark:
The wearing of artificial fingernails by medical staff must be refused. It has been documented in specialist literature that outbreaks of Pseudomonas aeruginosa, Candida, or ESBL-developing Klebsiella could be traced back to artificial fingernails[45].

Jewellery including watches and wedding rings is not allowed to be worn on the arm and forearm when engaged in activities which require a hygienic disinfection of the hands[46].

During disinfection of hands they must be kept moist throughout the required/prescribed exposure time.

If the hands get visibly contaminated during nursing activities, they shall be disinfected first and only be washed afterwards.

In case of contamination on a defined area of the hands they shall be cleaned first using a paper towel that has been soaked in disinfecting solution followed by disinfection and washing of hands.

---

[44] Mitteilung der Kommission für Krankenhaushygiene und Infektionsprävention am Robert-Koch-Institut: Händehygiene. Bundesgesundheitsbl. 2000 (43): 230-233

[45] HygMed 26, Jahrgang 2001

[46] BGR 250/TRBA 250 ch. 4.1.2.4

Heavily contaminated hands are an exception. In this case, the hands shall first be carefully rinsed off and then washed with warm water. The disinfection shall follow after drying off with paper towels.

A hygienic disinfection of the hands is necessary after contact with microbe-containing materials or contaminated objects and also after taking off gloves.
A hygienic disinfection of the hands has to be carried out for example:
- before taking up the nursing activity
- after every direct contact with patients
- before and after every contact with patients who are especially prone to infection e.g. immune-suppressed patients
- before preparation of injection solutions
- before setting up and connecting the dialysis lines and system
- before putting on gloves
- before every puncture
- before every manipulation at connection sites or vascular access
- before preparation and handling of drugs
- before entering the staff room
- before and after the preparation and distribution of food
- after contact with potentially or actually contaminated material, e.g. removal of bed-pans, disposal of wastes, etc.
- after use of the restroom or washroom
- after blowing the nose

Remark for the use of gloves:
In case of frequent change of gloves on one and the same patient, these gloves can be hygienically disinfected several times if they are not visibly contaminated [47, 48].
According to literature, some gloves can be disinfected several times with 60% Isopropanol without leaks appearing in the gloves. The success of disinfection

[47] Weber L. W.: Dichtigkeit von medizinischen Handschuhen unter Desinfektionsbelastung. In Dokumentationsband über die 39. Jahrestagung der Deutschen Gesellschaft für Arbeitsmedizin und Umweltmedizin, Hrsg. A. W. Retteneier und C. Feldhaus, Wiesbaden, 1999: 531-535

[48] DIN EN 455, Medizinische Handschuhe zum einmaligen Gebrauch

when wearing gloves was even better as with bare hands. This statement can however not be generalised for every type of glove. Disinfection is only acceptable when the disinfectability and the impermeability of a particular type of glove have been reproducibly tested. The recommendation to disinfect gloves in general and to use them on different patients shall be strictly rejected. In the daily routine, disinfection of the gloves can be practical and sensible in particular circumstances, e.g. reduction in the environmental contamination in intensive care units, if contamination took place during nursing activities in the course of which also components of devices or computer keyboards have to be touched. Similar rules apply in laboratories with contaminated material. Disinfection of gloves in case of infections (non-enveloped viruses!), direct blood contact or visible perforations shall always be rejected. In these cases, a careful disinfection of the hands and sufficient time to complete the drying of the skin shall be respected before putting on gloves again.
Authors of the literature state and suspect the problem is that in the daily routine, it cannot be expected that staff members have profound education on the problem in order to be able to recognise the limits of the above-mentioned procedures.
Disinfection of gloves in the clinical sector as a means of cost reduction is obsolete.

6.2.2 Skin Antiseptic

The skin is to be fully covered through spraying or application of the disinfectant. The skin is supposed to be kept moist with disinfectant during the exposure time according to the product information.
The following method shall be used when spraying: "spray – wipe off – spray". Sterile compresses for application, wiping and, if necessary, drying of the disinfectant shall be used when working on or close to native fistulas, prosthetic shunts and haemodialysis catheters.

6.2.3 Preparations (Disinfectants)

For hygienic disinfection of the hands and skin antisepsis, alcohol-based products shall be used due to the short exposure time. Only approved products and procedures and those listed by professional organisations have to be used which have at least a limited spectrum of virucidal activity and tuberculosity.

Editorial note:
According to a joint statement of the Robert Koch Institute (RKI), the German Society for Hygiene and Microbiology (DGHM), the German Association against Virus Diseases (DVV) and the German Society of Hygiene and Microbiology, there is a distinction between a virucidal and a limited virucidal activity. The term "limited virucidal", describes the activity against enveloped viruses e.g. HBV, HCV, HIV, while "virucidal" has an additional activity against non-enveloped viruses e.g. polio viruses, HAV, Norwalk-like viruses[49].

The presence of certain pathogens e.g. polio viruses, Norwalk-like viruses can require a longer exposure time and use of disinfectants listed by the RKI or classified as "virucidal".

Hand disinfectant containers must only be refilled under aseptic conditions in a pharmacy (German law)[50]. The use of disposable containers is advisable. Approved substances according to § 36 of the Arzneimittelgesetz/AMG (Pharmaceutical Act) can also be used.

6.2.4 Handling of Sterile Good Packaging and Sealing

Sterile goods have to be stored dry and in unopened or resealed packing in order to protect them from damage, dust, UV light and vermin. Sterile good packaging and sterile good sealing are to be opened only immediately before use. The expiry date and the integrity of the packaging have to be checked before use. The sterile goods taken out of the transport packaging have to be stored in closed drawers or cupboards. The principle of "first in, first out" applies for the storage and collection of sterile goods.

The storage requirements for sterile goods have to be respected in accordance with the DIN 58953 T8 and the instructions of the manufacturer.

[49] Prüfung und Deklaration der Wirksamkeit von Desinfektionsmitteln gegen Viren; Bundesgesundheitsblatt 2004 (47): 62-66, (www.rki.de)
[50] Arzneimittelgesetz § 4 Abs. 14, § 13, § 14, § 15

Type of Packaging	Storage	
	Unprotected[1]	Protected[2]
Primary package[3]	48 Hours	6 Months
Store package[4]	5 Years, insofar as there is no other expiry date fixed by the manufacturer	

[1] e.g. open drawers
[2] e.g. closed dust-free drawers and cupboards
[3] sealed or closed packaging system which surrounds the medical device completely sealing it off from germs (DIN EN 868-1:1997-05)
[4] package which contains one or more primary and/or secondary packages and which shall provide the necessary protection during long-term storage (DIN 58953-8:2003-10)

Tab. 1: Recommended period of storage for sterile medical devices according to DIN 58953-8:2003

Remark:
The time mentioned is to be considered as the maximum duration.

6.2.5 Surfaces

After every dialysis treatment, all potentially contaminated surfaces which come into contact with the hands and skin e.g. dialysis machines, work surfaces, sinks, water fittings, door handles, operating panel of single-place reverse osmosis units and other, are to be cleaned and disinfected using wipe/scrub disinfection. Details are to be checked for in the hygiene plan. Immediate disinfection is necessary after visible contamination of areas, technical equipment/machines, writing equipment, etc.

Disinfectants based on oxygen releasers shall not be applied because of their loss of effectiveness when exposed to blood. The use of alcoholic surface disinfectants may cause damage to certain plastic materials.

The disinfection shall be carried out with an approved substance and procedure using the 1-hour value concentration or higher concentration, if shorter exposure time is used. If higher concentration is recommended to inactivate hepatitis B, this concentration has to be chosen.

Visible contamination must first be wiped off using a wipe soaked with disinfectant. The procedure has to be repeated if necessary. The cleaned surface then needs to be wiped twice with a disinfectant solution. A new wipe which is sufficiently moistened must be used each time.

Editorial note: Used wipes may be considered as infected material.

Disinfection of the floor must take place only in sections where infectious patients and patients with resistant microbes are treated [51].

6.2.6 Inventory and Tableware

Dialysis-specific working materials, e.g. blood pressure cuffs with direct skin contact, tourniquets, and stethoscopes are to be disinfected at the end of each dialysis treatment; and immediately after contamination with blood or secretions.

A dish washer with an approved disinfection procedure e.g. thermo-disinfection is to be used for cleaning dishes. The procedure has to be checked routinely. A central reprocessing of tableware and dishes within the dialysis unit is acceptable when appropriate conditions are respected.

If no possibility of disinfecting dishes of infectious patients (thermal programme in machines > 93 °C/10 minutes) is available, disposables shall be used.

[51] RKI-Empfehlung: Anforderungen der Hygiene bei Reinigung und Desinfektion von Flächen. Bundesgesundheitsbl. – Gesundheitsforsch – Gesundheitsschutz 2004 (47): 51-61 (www.rki.de)

Books, journals and children's toys must be disinfected or disposed of after contamination with infectious materials.

6.2.7 Laundry

6.2.7.1 Requirements for Linen

Linen intended to be reused must be disinfectable. The linen to be used must be free from pathogenic micro-organisms.

Remark:
Specific and sufficient use of cleaning and disinfecting agents and adequate rinsing to eliminate allergy-causing components are to be ensured.

6.2.7.2 Procedures and Cleaning or Disinfecting Agents

Validated procedures and cleaning or disinfecting agents have to be used for processing. During transport and storage, the linen has to be packed in a way that contamination is avoided. Dirty and clean linen must be separated.

6.2.7.3 Laundry Requirements

Linen from dialysis treatment units can only be washed and cleaned in laundries which guarantee approved procedures in accordance with the requirements of hospital hygiene and the prevention of infections. They shall be hygienically monitored. These laundries are supposed to work in conformity with the RKI guideline. The contracting with commercial laundry operators shall be settled through written contracts[52].

[52] Anlage zu Ziffer 4.4.3 und 6.4 der Richtlinie Krankenhaushygiene und Infektionsprävention des RKI „Anforderungen der Hygiene an die Wäsche aus Einrichtungen des Gesundheitsdienstes, die Wäscherei und den Waschvorgang und Bedingungen für die Vergabe von Wäsche an gewerbliche Wäschereien", Bundesgesundheitsbl. 1995 (7), (www.rki.de)

Self-processing of the linen shall comply with the same requirements.

6.2.7.4 Change of Linen

As linen from dialysis treatment units might be microbiologically contaminated and improper handling within the unit can lead to a spread of infections, the linen shall be regularly changed. In ambulatory haemodialysis units it is acceptable that the linen, e.g. sheets, pillowcases and blankets used by individual patients are stored in individually allocated wardrobes in between the dialysis treatments. Linen shall be changed immediately if visibly contaminated, to latest by every fortnight or after being used 6-7 times, and sent off to an approved laundry. The individual linen wardrobes shall be cleaned with disinfecting wipe solution when the linen are changed.

During the change of used linen, attention needs to be paid to foreign materials in it. Dirty linen shall directly be placed into the appropriate linen basket. The linen baskets or containers, e.g. laundry bags are tightly sealed and stored in an appropriate room until their prompt transport to the laundry. Transport trolleys or containers have to be cleaned and disinfected after use. A hygienic disinfection of hands has to be carried out after disposing dirty linen.

6.2.7.5 Mattresses

Germ-proof protective covers, e.g. made of plastic foils impermeable to bacteria, mites and viruses are recommended for mattresses and have to undergo a wipe/scrub disinfection after each treatment. By covering the mattresses, central reprocessing by means of steam disinfection becomes dispensable.

6.2.7.6 Work Clothes[53]

The work clothes of nursing staff shall be changed daily. If there is any visible contamination, particular through blood, they have to be changed immediately. The employer is responsible for the disinfection and cleaning of contaminated working clothes.

6.2.7.7 Protective Clothing[54]

The employer has to provide a sufficient number of required protective clothing and other protective equipment at the disposal of employees. The protective clothing has to be worn over the work clothes. The employer is responsible for the regular disinfection, cleaning and maintenance of the protective clothing. Protective clothing and contaminated working clothes shall not be taken home by the employees.

6.2.7.8 Storage

There must be separate storage of clean linen and dirty linen. Contamination of the clean linen has to be excluded. It must also be ensured that there is no possible risk of contaminating the clean linen and working materials through the dirty linen. A hygienic disinfection of the hands has to be carried out before working with clean linen.

6.2.8 Reprocessing of Medical Devices in Dialysis

6.2.8.1 Introduction

The binding legal basis for the reprocessing of MP are § 3 of the Medical Devices Act (MPG) and § 4 of the "Medical Device Operator Ordinance" (MPBetreibV) which state that: "A proper

[53] BGR 250/TRBA 250, ch. 4.1.3
[54] BGR 250/TRBA 250, ch. 4.1.3

reprocessing is assumed when the joint recommendation of the Commission for Hospital Hygiene and Prevention of Infections at the Robert Koch Institute (RKI) and the Federal Institute for Drugs and Medical Devices are respected".

The key points of this joint recommendation from the RKI and the Federal Institute for Drugs and Medical Devices (BfArM) are specified in this guideline.[55]

The operator of a facility is supposed to entrust the servicing (e.g. maintenance, inspection, repairs, and reprocessing) of medical devices only to persons, companies or facilities who have the expertise, preconditions and required means to properly execute the task.

When reprocessing[56] microbe-reduced or sterile medical devices which are supposed to be used sterile instructions of the manufacturer must be strictly followed and validated procedures used. The outcome of these procedures must meet the defined requirements and the health of patients, users and others shall not be endangered. Instructions for use or user's manual of every medical device must be available.

Particular care shall be taken to ensure that the use of reprocessed medical device poses no risk e.g.:

- **infections**
- **pyrogenic-induced reactions**
- **allergic reactions**
- **toxic reactions**
- **malfunctioning due to altered technical and functional characteristics**

[55] Anforderungen an die Hygiene bei der Aufbereitung von Medizinprodukten. Bundesgesundheitsbl – Gesundheitsforsch – Gesundheitsschutz, 2001 (44): 1115-1126 (www.rki.de)

[56] R. Hill, J.M. Schmitt, WiKo Medizinproduktrecht Kommentar, Verlag Dr. Otto Schmidt KG, Köln

The essential constructive and functional features which are responsible for the security and operational efficiency have to be examined after maintenance or repairs of medical devices as far as they can be influenced by the maintenance measures.

The implementation of the "requirements on hygiene during the reprocessing of medical devices" shall be easier in hospital dialysis centres as they can rely on the central sterilisation unit of the hospital. For ambulatory dialysis facilities without access to a central sterilisation unit it can be recommended to use sterile single use material instead. When reprocessing medical devices they shall not go beyond classification "Critical A" class.

A violation of § 4 of the Medical Device Operator Ordinance (MPBetreibV) can be penalised with a fine and in serious cases even be classified as a statutory offence.

6.2.8.2 Field of application

The requirements apply to products or parts of products, including accessories, which are meant to

- be brought into contact with the human body or
- be inserted in the human body
- blood, blood elements, other body fluids or body tissue
  - to lead through
  - to change in their composition or
  - to store for later use on human beings

Furthermore, products and parts of products (including accessories) are recorded that aid to induce gas and other preparations into the human body for the purpose of:

- infusion
- reinfusion
- perfusion or
- other application or induction

6.2.8.3 Quality Assurance

A quality management system which makes use of the recognised rules of the technique (RKI guideline, standards) or the state of science and technology is necessary in order to comply with the hygiene requirements needed for the reprocessing of medical devices. It is advisable to document the organisation of reprocessing of medical devices in the hygiene plan.

Following steps shall be taken:

a) Risk assessment of the medical device to be processed
b) Classification into risk groups (see table in ch. 6.2.8.6) in accordance with the RKI guideline
c) Definition of responsibilities for all the steps of the reprocessing
d) Detailed description (standard operating procedures) of the practical execution of procedures to be used and of necessary examinations
e) Regular instruction of staff responsible for the reprocessing of medical devices.

Rights and duties of contractors and customers as well as the modalities for the transportation and return of medical devices shall be regulated in writing when the reprocessing is performed by an outside contractor. The contractor shall provide evidence of a certified quality management system (QMS).

The QMS has to be certified according to EN ISO 13485 or 13488 in case of especially stringent requirements for reprocessing (medical devices of "critical C" group).

If manual cleaning and disinfection procedures are used

- documented standard operating procedures must be available
- the effectiveness of the procedures must be validated
- they must be adapted to each medical device

In case of automated reprocessing following procedures have to be carried out:

- start-up testing
- daily routine testing
- batch-related routine testing
- meteorological monitoring and inspection of the procedural parameters
- periodic testing

Remark:
The working group takes up the position that the necessary measurable monitoring, inspection, batch-related documentation and release according to the RKI guideline apply only for medical devices of the classification "critical". A semi-annual inspection using biological indicators shall be sufficient for bed-pan cleaning devices (cleaning and disinfection); cleaning and disinfection automates in which exclusively clamps for shunt compression are prepared.

6.2.8.4 Risk Assessment

It is to be checked before the reprocessing
- whether
- with which procedure
- if applicable how often and
- under which conditions (rooms, working material, and qualification of staff) medical devices have to be processed and stored.

Critical steps during the procedure and potential risks have to be defined for the necessary measures of risk minimisation.

6.2.8.5 Risks

Depending on previous use, further utilisation, composition of the medical device and the reprocessing procedure used the following aspects have to be taken into consideration:
- Type and quantity of the pathogen to be expected
- Resistance of the pathogen regarding the specific reprocessing procedure

- Possible risks caused by undesired effects due to
  - residues resulting from previous use (e.g. blood and its components, secretions, medicine)
  - residues resulting from previous reprocessing procedures (e.g. cleaning agents, disinfectants and sterilising agents)
  - residues from other agents including their reaction products
- Transport and storage
- Type of subsequent use
- Risks caused by changes in the physical, chemical or functional characteristics of the medical device
- Risks through altered composition of the materials
  - accelerated deterioration of materials
  - embrittlement
  - altered surface characteristics
  - alterations of contact sites and adhesive connection sites

6.2.8.6 Measures

Manufacturers of medical devices have to provide the following information about the reprocessing procedure

- cleaning and disinfection
- rinsing
- drying
- packaging
- sterilisation
- transport
- appropriate storage

Deviations are tolerable if they are justified and documented. The functional ability to meet the purpose and to complete guarantee for safety of use must not be restricted. The applied procedure requires testing and validation.

Content of Standard Working Conditions for the Reprocessing of Medical Devices

Remark:
For a better understanding, it is necessary to clearly explain what is to be legally understood when the term reprocessing is used. According to § 3, N° 14 of the Medical Products Act (MPG) the reprocessing of medical devices encompasses cleaning, disinfection and sterilisation including the related stages of work as well as the examination and restoration of the functional technological security (legal definition). If the medical devices are only cleaned and/or disinfected it is a matter of repairs. The term maintenance[57] in contrast encompasses the servicing, repairs and preparation. In line with this interpretation, it is the maintenance of medical devices which usually takes place in dialysis.[58]

a) Collecting used Medical Devices and transportation to the Reprocessing site

When collecting and transporting medical devices to a reprocessing site contamination of the environment must be excluded. Collecting and transportation shall take place immediately after use, in containers with smooth, easy to clean and disinfectant-resistant surfaces. Dry transport shall be carried out as far as possible. Medical devices shall be drained before disposal as much as possible. Dialysis machines shall preferably be reprocessed at the treatment site.

b) Execution of the Cleaning

For this procedure, internal and external surfaces must be accessible in order to avoid cross-contamination and impairment of safety of use and guarantee the absence of residues.

If possible, alkaline agents shall be used, because in contact with fat and protein residues they exhibit a good cleaning performance and have an antimicrobial effect.

[57] MPBetreibV § 4

[58] R. Hill, J.M. Schmitt WiKo WiKo Medizinprodukterecht Kommentar, Verlag Dr. Otto Schmidt KG, Köln

Changing the cleansing solution once a day in cleansing baths is sufficient – in case of any visible contamination, the solution shall be changed immediately.

The cleansing basin has to be mechanically cleaned and disinfected daily.

c) Execution of Disinfection

The disinfection procedure must encompass the A B activity spectrum, i.e.

- fungicidal
- bactericidal
- virucidal, but at least be effective for HBV

There shall be no risk of infection in case of skin and/or mucosa contact with the medical device. Thermal procedures are preferable. Residues from disinfectants shall not be fixated. If possible, no alcohol or aldehyde shall be used when sterilisation has to be performed afterwards.

When organising the work routines following has to be respected:

- the instructions for use
- the intended purpose
- the concentration
- the exposure time of the disinfectant
- the procedural steps

Reactive products and residues can be avoided by sufficient rinsing with water of appropriate quality. Re-contamination shall be avoided.

d) Inspection of Functional and Technical Safety

The accountability is with the operator. Thus, simple functional inspections relevant for the safety of the medical device shall be carried out before sterilisation and immediately before use.

e) Packaging

Mechanical protective packaging, sterile packaging and repackaging must be aligned with:

- the sterilisation procedure
- the preservation of special characteristics and the functional ability of the medical device
- the storage and transport

f) Sterilisation

The success of the sterilisation depends on:

- the accuracy of the cleaning
- the suitability of the (validated) procedure
- the packaging
- the loading of the sterilisers

g) Labelling

Labelling of the sterilised products is necessary:

- to differentiate whether it is released
- as information about time-dependent aspects of safe use and storage deadlines

If the reprocessing is done by a third party, the name and address must be mentioned on the packaging. Furthermore limitations regarding the number of allowed sterilisation processes must be respected. It must be obvious to the user whether the conditioning process ends with the sterilisation or with the disinfection.

h) Release of Sterilised Goods

The reprocessing ends with the release of the goods for use. This release includes:

- the performance and documentation of the daily inspection routine
- the inspection and documentation of the complete and correct course of the process
- the inspection of the packaging if necessary
- the inspection of the labelling if necessary

The persons authorised to release products are to be named in writing. As long as only medical devices up till class "A-critical" are exclusively being dealt with, this naming becomes unnecessary in the ambulatory dialysis units, as this belongs to the job profile of every qualified nurse and formally educated medical assistant to process these types of medical devices.
The standard working condition also contains the form of documentation of the release decision as well as the procedure to follow if there are deviations from the correct course of the process.

i) Documentation

The registered measurements [e.g. temperature, time, pressure (in autoclaves)] and the release decision with reference to the releasing person and the batch have to be documented and stored when dealing with disinfection automates and sterilisation machines.
The storage period for this documentation is 5 years (following § 9 of the Medical Device Operator Ordinance – MPBetreibV).

j) Transportation and Storage

The medical device is not supposed to experience any disadvantageous influences through transportation and storage. The instructions of the manufacturer of the medical device are to be respected as well as those of the manufacturer of the packaging material.
During transportation and storage the product must be protected from:
- mechanical influences
- dust

- humidity
- UV light
- heat
- vermin

Criteria for the risk classification of medical devices and requirements for their reprocessing

Classification	Medical devices	Examples	Critical Procedural Steps/ Special Requirements
Uncritical	Contact with healthy skin	Fistula clamps, blood pressure cuff, ECG-electrode, tourniquet, blood line clamp, bedpan, stethoscope, ultrasonic transducer	Disinfection with certified procedures
Semi-critical **A)** without special requirements	Contact with the mucosa or pathologically altered skin surface	Thermometer, mandrill, intubation spatula, Magill's forceps, mouth prop, oxygen masks, urine bottle, tubus	Disinfection with certified products/ procedures (AB activity spectrum according to the definition of the RKI list).
B) with special requirements		Respiratory mask, resuscitation tube, dialysis machine, oral airway, tracheal tube	Number of applications or reprocessing cycles are defined by the manufacturer. The success of cleaning cannot be immediately determined through inspection. The reprocessing can influence the use and functionality. Preferably automated cleaning and disinfection.
Critical **A)** without special requirements	Use of blood, blood products and sterile medical products. Penetration of the skin or mucosa, contact with blood, internal tissues including wounds.	Scissors (for non-invasive purposes), scalpel, forceps	Preferably machine cleaning and disinfection; steam sterilisation
B) with increased requirements		Suction catheter, blood lines, tubing system, cannulas, buttonhole probe, scissors (for invasive purposes), syringes, titanium adapters	Reprocessing or number of reprocessing cycles is limited by the manufacturer. The success of cleaning cannot be immediately determined. Reprocessing can influence use and safety of the functionality. In addition: Proof of recognised professional education as a sterile goods assistant who is entrusted with the reprocessing
C) with particularly high requirements	+ thermo-sensitive medical devices to be used invasively	Dialysers	Medical devices that do not tolerate steam of 134 °C sterilisation. External quality control Proof of certified QMS through an office accredited by the responsible authority. Risk analysis according to DIN EN ISO 14971

Remark: Bed-pans and urine bottles are to be classified as medical devices only when they are used exclusively for medical purposes. Otherwise they are considered as products which help in facilitating daily life – i.e. articles or objects of daily use.

6.2.9 Reuse

Disposable medical products like dialysers and blood lines for example are for single use. Therefore, the reuse of dialysers and blood line systems shall be refused at present.
If they are reprocessed despite of the associated risks, this procedure must comply with the requirements of the Medical Device Act.
This can only be allowed when it is guaranteed that the product is being reused on the same patient only. Risks involved are: loss of quality with regards to the characteristics of the material, formation of coats on the surface of the material, obstructions, insufficient sterilisation or disinfection, chemical denaturalised protein residues, and reduced clearance. The impact and costs make reprocessing impracticable for the practitioner.

6.2.10 Use of Disinfectants and Cleaning Agents

6.2.10.1 Handling of Hazardous Substances

Disinfectants or cleaning agents are mostly called "dangerous preparations"[59]. They can be harmful to health if not used adequately. Gloves, safety glasses and protective clothing are supposed to be worn at all times when handling these preparations.
Detailed information can be taken from the information for use or the safety data sheets of the product. Particular attention shall be paid to the fact that products shall not be mixed as this could possibly lead to dangerous reactions and be harmful to health. In addition, the antimicrobial power could be neutralised.

6.2.10.2 Safe Application

In order to guarantee the success of the disinfection, it is important to apply the correct dosage of disinfectant and respect the exposure time.

[59] GefahrstoffV § 3

The bactericidal and/or veridical effect is not guaranteed when an insufficient dosage is used. As a consequence micro-organisms might develop resistance and thus can spread within the facility.

Incorrect high dosages can lead to material damages or health risks, e.g. higher evaporation of aldehyde-containing disinfectants due to the stronger concentration of active agents.

6.2.10.3 Safe Use

Regarding the handling of hazardous substances, local conditions as well as the safety data sheets have to be considered.

For the greatest possible safety to be guaranteed, the following points among others are to be observed:

- Safety advice in the information for use
- Ensure ventilation during the use of surface disinfectants (especially when dealing with aldehyde preparations)
- Never work without chemical-proof gloves, e.g. household gloves when using surface and instrument disinfectants
- Always tightly seal and safely store containers after use
- Removing possibly leaked-out disinfectants taking into consideration the danger of inflammation
- Always keep disinfection tubs used for manual disinfection of instruments closed with a lid
- Never mix different disinfectants (danger of chemical reactions, e.g. the release of chloric gas)
- Storage on acid-resistant floors
- Storage of different hazardous substances in spatial distances e.g. different tubs
- Containers must be completely emptied before being disposed of

Remark:
Due to safety and technical reasons, alcohol preparations are not suitable for extensive surface disinfection (inflammable, aerosol formation, inhalation risks).

6.2.10.4 Requirements on the Manufacturers

The manufacturer is supposed to supply information about "dangerous substances" supplying specifications in the information for use and on the safety data sheets.

6.2.10.5 Requirements on the Employer and User[60]

Risk evaluation concerning the working conditions shall be done by a professional before work can be started with hazardous substances. The employer has to procure the necessary information, e.g. safety data sheets which are needed to carry out the evaluation of the danger. The employer has to set up safety measures and operating instructions for the handling of these working substances based on this information. The operating instructions have to be displayed.

These operating instructions can also be obtained directly from the manufacturer in the form of instruction templates.

Before starting work with dangerous substances users have to be instructed and then regularly educated. The user must follow the instructions and adhere to the security measures.

6.2.11 Dispatch of Diagnostic Samples

Special packaging and dispatching conditions have to be observed when dispatching diagnostic samples. If the dispatching is done per post, the transportation conditions are to be observed[61].

---

[60] GefahrstoffV § 3

[61] RKI: Neue Bestimmungen zur Beförderung ansteckungsgefährlicher Stoffe. Epidemiologisches Bulletin 2005 (4)

6.3 Water and Solutions for Haemodialysis Procedures

6.3.1 Drinking Water

The Drinking Water Ordinance (TrinkwV) is valid right up to the transfer point of the supply pipe of the water supply company or the domestic installation to the water purification plant of the dialysis unit as well as with regards to controls.

The chlorine content of drinking water must continuously be < 0.1 ppm otherwise an appropriate activated carbon filter for the elimination of chlorine has to be installed in the purification unit between the softener and reverse osmosis.

An agreement has to be reached with the water supply company according to which the dialysis unit will be informed about planned or already carried out chlorinating measures.

Remark:
The water supply companies are normally ready to provide information about their water quality. However, an obligation of the water supply company to directly inform the dialysis unit does not exist. Therefore the operator has to ask for information which is important for the procedures carried out in the dialysis unit (s. ch. 11.4: Letter to Communal Water Suppliers).

6.3.2 Permeate

Permeate used for diluting concentrated haemodialysis solutions is produced from drinking water by means of a reverse osmosis unit. The conditions for manufacturing, transportation/distribution and storage have to be selected so that the risk of a chemical and/or microbial contamination is kept low. To determine the chemical quality, the regulations of the European Pharmacopoeia[62] (Ph. Eur.)

[62] Europäisches Arzneibuch 4. Ausgabe, Grundwerk 2002: 1167: Wasser zum Verdünnen konzentrierter Hämodialyselösung. Editorial note: update of European Pharmacopoeia 6th Edition 2008

in the form valid at the time are to be used while the regulations of the RKI are to be consulted in order to determine the microbiological quality. The working group recommends the regulations of the Association for the Advancement of Medical Instrumentation (AAMI) to be taken into consideration for missing parameters/critical values in the regulations of the Ph. Eur (see table ch. 11.3).

Remark:
Monographs for haemodialysis solutions and haemodialysis concentrates and for water used in diluting concentrated haemodialysis solutions can be found in the European Pharmacopoeia.
(Editorial note: New international standard is ISO 13959:2009 "Water for haemodialysis and related therapies")

6.3.3 Concentrates for Haemodialysis

Whether in centralised concentrate delivery systems (CDS), canisters, pouches, or cartouches, the connection of the concentrate must be carried out under defined hygienic conditions and specifically described in the hygiene plan.

Remark:
Dialysis concentrates are medical devices.
(Editorial note: New international standard is ISO 13958:2009 "Concentrates for haemodialysis and related therapies")

6.3.4 Dialysis Fluids

Dialysis fluids (permeate + haemodialysis concentrate(s)) are electrolyte solutions with a concentration which is almost equal to the electrolyte concentration of normal extracellular body fluid (plasma). The solutions can contain glucose.

(Editorial note: New international standard is ISO 11663:2009 "Quality of dialysis fluid for haemodialysis and related therapies")

6.3.5 Substitution Fluids for Online Procedures

On-line procedures are described as blood cleaning procedures which use dialysis fluid specially prepared through additional filtration steps to make them suitable for use as infusion/substitutive fluids. At the same time the chemical composition can be determined through the appropriate choice ad dosage of haemodialysis concentrates and permeates. The microbiological purity is guaranteed through so-called ultra filters and appropriate disinfection measures.

The administered infusion, e.g. volume of 10-70 litres per 4 hour treatment, must be sterile and free of pyrogens.

Remark:
Formally, the process is equal to professional production of a medicinal product by the responsible physician. The courses and requirements on the production process in terms of equipment are validated by the manufacturers of the equipment. They are subject to the same quality requirements like infusions and, therefore, legally fall under the remarks of the Medicines Act (AMG) and they must be in conformity with the requirements of the European Pharmacopoeia. The device manufacturers are defining the conditions of use and the measures for quality assurance.

6.4 Monitoring and Evaluation of Permeate and Dialysis Fluids

All the points listed shall be described in the hygiene plan of the dialysis unit.

6.4.1 Handling Samples

The education of the staff on handling, taking and transporting samples can be done by anybody who is working in the interest of the instructed and delegating person who at the end assesses the result and proposes or orders measures.

6.4.2 Collecting Samples

The collection of samples has to take place at defined sampling points and under aseptic conditions. Precise working instructions have to be defined and documented of the sample collection. Any equipment used in taking samples for identification of endotoxin must be free of endotoxin and shall not be able to absorb endotoxin (instructions of the laboratory concerning transportation shall be respected if necessary).

6.4.3 Transportation

Samples taken for viable count shall be processed within 24 hours and samples taken for the identification of pyrogens within a maximum of 48 hours. After collecting the samples they have to be stored in a refrigerator until they are picked up. The required storage temperature of 4 °C needs to be maintained during transportation and according to the instructions of the examining laboratory.

6.4.4 Scope of Analysis

The microbiological analysis encompasses:

- identification of living and growing microbes (colony-forming units = cfu/ml)
- identification of Pseudomonas aeruginosa per 100 ml
  (Editorial note: Special recommendations for Pseudomonas aeruginosa and Escherichia coli apply in some countries)

6.4.5 Viable Count[63]

In this guideline, the working group considers that germs found in water are better to detect at 22 °C than at 30-35 °C[64] and on appropriate culture media

(Editorial note: New international standards are ISO 13959:2009 "Water for haemodialysis and related therapies" and ISO 11663:2009 "Quality of dialysis fluid for haemodialysis and related therapies")

Volume of the sample	250 ml (1 ml out of this for measure of the total viable count), residual volume as far as needed for differentiation)
Procedure:	Suffusion or surface procedures/plating procedures
Substrates:	TGEA (Oxoid N° CM 0127), R2A
Incubation temperature:	22 °C ± 2 °C
Incubation period:	Evaluation after 3 and 7 days
Result:	cfu/1 ml after 7 days
Limit according to RKI:	100 cfu/ml
Warning limit (only after disinfection):	25 cfu/ml[65]

Remark: The limit of ≤ 10 cfu/ml to be complied with the European Pharmacopoeia is decisive. (Editorial note: ISO 13959:2009 and 11663:2009 define "incubation temperature at 17-23 °C" and general "action limit" at 50 cfu/ml)

[63] Ledebo I., Nystrand R.: Defining the microbiological quality of dialysis fluid. Artificial Organs 1999 (Jan 23 (1)), 37-43

[64] EDTNA/ERCA Guidelines: Technical Section. EDTNA/ERCA Journal 2002 (XXVIII-3): 119-129 (www.edtnaerca.org)

[65] EDTNA/ERCA Guidelines: Technical Section. EDTNA/ERCA Journal 2002 (XXVIII-3): 119-129 (www.edtnaerca.org)

6.4.6 Analysis of Pseudomonas aeruginosae[66]

Procedure:	membrane filtration or fluid enrichment
Substrates:	on selective culture mediums
Incubation temperature:	36 ± 1 °C
Incubation period:	at least 24 hrs
Result:	positive/negative/100 ml
Limit:	< 1 cfu/100 ml

Remark:
In order to obtain results which are comparable to the above-mentioned standards, the operator shall inform the laboratory of the microbiological methods suggested by this working group and the examinations shall be carried out following these methods[67].

6.4.7 Recommended Sampling Points

Sampling point 1	Transfer point from the water treatment plant or concentrate supply system to the beginning of the distribution pipes.
Sampling points 2 + 3	In the middle and at the end of each distribution pipe. In case of multiple floors one additional sample of each of the distribution pipes per floor.

Remark:
Additional sampling points if deemed necessary are to be determined by the responsible physician and/or the hospital hygienist.

[66] Recommended according to RKI: Anlage zur Richtlinie für Krankenhaushygiene und Infektionsprävention (www.rki.de)

[67] Nystrand, R.: Standards and standardisation of detection methods for bacteria and endotoxin in water and dialysis fluid, Nieren- und Hochdruckerkrankungen 1999; 28: 43-48

6.4.8 Sampling Schedule

The sampling for permeate for microbiological examination must take place:

a) 5-7 days after installation, initiation and disinfection
   5-7 days after disinfection, in case of modifications, i.e. after intervention on the pipe system supplying permeate or liquid bicarbonate concentrates
b) In case of deterioration of the microbiological quality of the drinking water
c) At least every six months
d) In case of patient reactions due to potential microbiological causes in the fluid supply system
e) 5-7 days after disinfection due to exceeding the limit or warning limit

(Editorial note: Depending on the design and disinfection strategy of the permeate, dialysis concentrate and dialysis fluid system the provider has the right to decide upon alternative actions)

6.4.9 Endotoxin Analysis

In addition to the microbiological examination every 6 months an annual endotoxin analysis is recommended.
Endotoxin analysis shall also be done in special cases such as

- starting up of a new water treatment plant
- evaluation of pyrogenic reactions

Procedure:	Gel-Clot; chromogenic; turbidimetric
Result:	data in IU/ml
Limit:	< 0.25 IU/ml

Remark:
The endotoxin test cannot replace the total viable count[68, 69].

[68] EDTNA/ERCA Guidelines: Technical Section. EDTNA/ERCA Journal 2002 (XXVIII-3): 119-129, (www.edtnaerca.org)

[69] Nystrand, R.: Can endotoxin testing replace microbiological cultivation? Abstract book 2005, p. 42, 10th annual conference of the Japanese Society of Haemodiafiltration

(Editorial note: ISO 11663:2009 has the limit for dialysis fluid of < 0.5 EU/ml and ultra pure dialysis fluid < 0.03 EU/ml.)

6.4.10 Examination for Fungal Contamination

It is recommended to annually check the presence of fungi in the central supply systems for concentrates[70].

6.4.11 Evaluation of Results

The evaluation of results has to be performed by a competent laboratory.

Remark:
Long-term recording and evaluation by the provider is useful in terms of quality assurance.

6.5 Disinfection Measures for the Fluid Pathway and the Dialysis Machines

6.5.1 General

The reverse osmosis unit and the water distribution system are to be jointly considered in terms of hygienic aspects. The manufacturer or supplying or installation companies of single components within a complete system are obliged to describe effective disinfection procedures for the complete system installed. If system components of different manufacturers/suppliers are combined, the operator in agreement with the manufacturers has to guarantee that this specific combination of single components will still allow safe production, distribution and disinfection procedures[71].

[70] EDTNA/ERCA Guidelines: Technical Section. EDTNA/ERCA Journal 2002 (XXVIII-3): 119-129, (www.edtnaerca.org)
[71] MPG § 3 Abs. 15

The concentration of the disinfectant, for example, has to be measured at the point of collection, drainage and return of permeate. The required exposure times have to be monitored at every site. For thermal procedures, the minimum temperature has to be measured in the return or at the most peripheral point.

6.5.2 Dialysis Machines

Between treatments and after service measurers the dialysis machine has to be cleaned and disinfected following the instructions of the manufacturer. Additional dialysis machines shall be used daily in a so called rotation-scheme so that each machine is regularly integrated in the therapeutical cycle. In case of a longer period out of use, the machine must be disinfected before use according to the manufacturer's guidelines.

The dialysis machines have to be processed (chemically, chemothermally or thermally) with validated disinfection procedures.

The machine manufacturer or distributor has to supply suitable validated disinfection procedures for his special type of machine. These specifications must contain information on the methods to be used for checking on residuals of disinfectant. Verification method must show specific sensitivity to detect any residues in the hydraulic circuit, in order to prevent any possible harm to patients. The release of the dialysis machine for next treatment can only take place when the absence of any disinfectant residues has been tested and appropriately documented.

The disinfection procedures must comply with these guidelines and have to be incorporated in the hygiene plan of the dialysis centre.

Since nurses and patients are present in the treatment room during the work cycle no unreasonable offensive smells or irritations of the respiratory tract shall be produced during disinfection[72].

The disinfectants and disinfecting agents used shall cause as little pollution as possible when introduced into the public water waste system. The local requirements for water discharge have to be respected[73].

6.5.3 Re-introduction of a Dialysis Machine from a Section with Blood Transmissible Viral Infections

Without exact proof, the members of the working group consider that the transmission of viruses especially hepatitis viruses can occur in dialysis units in the following order of priority:

- via hands
- via surfaces of the machines and
- via the interior water leading pathway of the dialysis machines

Though the danger of transmission through the dialysis machines is the least likely, without proper disinfection it cannot be excluded. Validated disinfection procedures minimise these risks in the re-introduction of machines from patients with blood transmissible viral infections into the normal cycle of use in the unit.

The reprocessing of a "yellow" to a "white" machine shall be an exceptional case.

Two successive procedures for the hydraulic system of the machine have to be used:

1. Step: Decalcification and disinfection (acidic disinfectant)
2. Step: Cleaning and disinfection (alkaline disinfectant)

---

[72] GefahrstoffV § 7

[73] Wasserhaushaltsgesetz

Reasons:

Viruses can be covered by calcareous residues, proteins and fats and therefore protected and present in the machine. In order to guarantee safe decalcification or cleaning of the contaminated machine, a two-step procedure has to be carried out always using an approved disinfectant.

For special cases in which a so-called "yellow" dialysis machine has to be reprocessed, the proposed procedure has to be ordered in writing by the medical management of the dialysis treatment unit. Only machines on which the above-mentioned disinfection procedures are applicable are allowed to be transferred for the use in the non-infectious patient section. The execution of the procedure must be monitored by an authorised and instructed person and documented in a disinfection protocol (s. ch. 11.5). The protocol has to be signed by two persons (the physician in charge and supervision nurse) to make sure that in this case, the reprocessing does not take place routinely but is done with increased attention.

A change of the sterile filter is recommended by the machine manufacturers.

Changing of the pressure transducer is not required. The pressure transducer shall always be immediately changed if there is suspicion of a contamination (passing blood/plasma through the contamination barrier/hydrophobic filter).

Changing of the dialysis machine coupling is not required. They shall be included in the intensive surface disinfection process.

The procedure used for standard haemodialysis machines applies also to the so-called online machines.

6.5.4 Disinfection of Central Permeate Supplying Systems

If a regular thermal disinfection is not possible due to the material used for the piping system, the supply system can be chemically disinfected and cleaned depending on the defined/set quality objectives of the centre. In this case all the manufacturers' instructions for performing such a disinfection for the complete supply system have to be followed, considering the disinfectants, procedures and evaluation processes to be used.

Preventive disinfection shall not be carried out in old installations when values/viable count do/does not exceed the defined limits.

Remark:
The biofilm which is stable up till the chemical disinfection will only be partially removed. That is why increased viable colony and endotoxin values, which can only be kept under control through repeated disinfection, must be expected[74].

6.5.4.1 Sanitation

Sanitation is required after repeatedly exceeding the critical value and unsuccessful disinfection measures in contaminated supply systems. It is performed on empirical basis and depending on the length of the supply system, the construction material and most importantly the microflora in the piping systems; different procedures will have to be combined. Regular disinfection for the maintenance of the microbiological quality is required after successful sanitation. The required microbiological quality determines further measures.

A performance review after 5-7 days, a bacteriological analysis as well as an analysis of endotoxin and a follow-up examination during three successive months is recommended.

[74] EDTNA/ERCA Guidelines: Technical Section. EDTNA/ERCA Journal 2002 (XXVIII-3): 119-129, (www.edtnaerca.org)

6.5.4.2 Interventions in the System

Disinfection accompanied by a performance review of the viable colony count and endotoxin is necessary after interventions in the permeate-conducting system. The required microbiological quality determines further measures.

Remark:
The realisation of the work on the permeate-conducting system is to be carried out under hygienic aspects. Technicians must first disinfect their hands and possibly put on gloves during plumbing.

6.5.4.3 Freedom from Disinfectants

After disinfection, cleaning and rinsing, the freedom of chemicals must be guaranteed by using suitable measures in order to avoid causing any dangers to the patients, e.g. through insufficiently washed out feeding pipes.

6.5.5 Concentrate Supply Systems (Bicarbonate and Acid Concentrate)

New supply systems for concentrates shall be provided with a possibility of disinfection. Central bicarbonate concentrate supply without preventive disinfection is to be rejected due to the high risk of germ growth. Acid concentrate ring pipes show a limited risk of microbial contamination. Nevertheless, there shall be the possibility of disinfecting the system in order to be able to treat possible flora of mould[75] for example.

[75] EDTNA/ERCA Guidelines: Technical Section. EDTNA/ERCA Journal 2002 (XXVIII-3): 119-129 (www.edtnaerca.org)

7 Particular Aspects of Hygiene in Dialysis Treatment

7.1 Vascular access

7.1.1 Goal and Rationale

- Prevention of bacterial contamination, infection and sepsis of the vascular access
- Prevention of infection-related loss of vascular access, in order to avoid hospitalisation and costs for intervention, reconstruction, antibiosis
- Prevention of cross-contamination

Infections are the second most common cause of death among patients with end-stage renal disease (ESRD)[76] following cardiovascular incidents. They can be reduced by applying focused and comprehensive hygienic working routines in handling of vascular access. Handling of the vascular access (for dialysis treatment) must be very careful and hygienically appropriate since this influences directly the quality of treatment as well as quality of life and life expectancy of patients[77].
Continuous assessment and evaluation, identifications of complications, traceable documentation, and information of the physician shall take place regularly.

7.1.2 Definition

Vascular access for haemodialysis and related extracorporeal therapies are native arterio-venous (AV) fistula, grafts, central venous

[76] Quasi-Niere: Nierenersatztherapie in Deutschland. Bericht über Dialysebehandlung und Nierentransplantation in Deutschland 20032004 (www.quasi-niere.de)

[77] National Kidney Foundation. K/DOQI Clinical Practice Guidelines for Vascular Access, 2000. Am J Kidney Dis 37: 137-187, 2001 (suppl 1), (www.kidney.org)

catheters with soft or stiff tip, implanted atrial catheters (CVC), and port systems.

Remark: The terms "shunt" and "fistula" are equivalent.

7.1.3 Qualification and Assignment

All the staff handling vascular access must be educated regularly since it is documented that educated staff is (more) effective in preventing and reducing contamination and infection rate in vascular access and central catheters[78, 79].
The number of patients treated by one nurse (together with the supporting nursing assistants) shall be limited considering structural and organisational circumstances to ensure safe and complication-free care. A drastic increase of incidents and errors in handling vascular access as well as in the resulting costs has to be expected when these limits are exceeded[80].

7.1.4 Creation of Vascular Access

During the creation of vascular access hygienic requirements must comply with general hygienic standards as applied in the operation theatre department[81]. The principles of surgical wound care must be applied.
The extent of the tissue trauma during catheter insertion can influence survival time of the CVC.

[78] RKI-Empfehlung: Prävention Gefäßkatheter-assoziierter Infektionen. Bundesgesundheitsbl. – Gesundheitsforsch – Gesundheitsschutz, 2002 (45): 907-924 (www.rki.de)

[79] National Kidney Foundation. K/DOQI Clinical Practice Guidelines for Vascular Access, 2000. Am J Kidney Dis 37: 137-187, 2001 (suppl. 1) (www.kidney.org)

[80] Elseviers, M.M., Lindley, E.J. van Waeleghem, J.P.: Management of the vessel inlet in Europe Part 1, EDTNA/ERCA Journal XXVI, 2000 (4): 29-35

[81] Raad, I.I. et al.: Prevention of central venous catheter-related infections by using maximal sterile barrier precautions during insertion. Infection Control and Hospital Epidemiology, 1994 (15 (4)): 231-238

The tension-free, secure fixation of the CVC after initial placement can influence the catheter's survival time positively.

7.1.5 Handling of AV Fistula

Vascular access for haemodialysis shall be handled only by trained and educated staff. The access is established only for the single purpose of dialysis treatment.

Procedure

- Hygienic hand disinfection must be carried out before shunt puncturing.
- Disposable gloves must be worn during the puncture.
- In order to prevent auto-infection (especially Staphylococcus aureus from the nose), the needling nurse and patient shall wear a mask to cover mouth and nose and the patient's face shall be turned away.
- The puncturing nurse and patient shall not speak during the process of setting or correcting the needles.
- Washing of the area of needle placement is only recommended if there is visible contamination. Water residue on the skin after washing can dilute the disinfectant and limit the efficacy of the disinfection procedure.
- The skin disinfection procedure must be carried out taking into account the exposure time. "Wet or spray-wet" disinfection shall be carried out twice using sterile compresses in between.
- Depending on the patients, spray or liquid disinfectants shall be used as spray or fluid.
  Remark:
  When using sprays, aerosols can have a bronchi-toxic effect on patients and staff[82].
- Sterile material must be used to cover the puncture sites.

[82] BGR 206: Desinfektionsarbeiten im Gesundheitsdienst (www.bgw-online.de)

- For further fixation of blood lines distant from the puncture sites hygienic dressing can be used. Sterile dressing must be used for fixation close to the puncture site.
- Each patient shall be given her/his own tourniquet.
- For compression of puncture site the patient shall use disposable gloves to avoid smear infections due to blood contaminated fingers and hands.
- Fistula clamps shall be cleaned and disinfected after each use.

Remark:
The facility has a defined and described safe procedure for the protection of the shunt function.

7.1.6 Grafts (Prosthetic Shunts, CVC and Port Systems)

Prosthetic shunts, CVCs and ports are exposed to an increased risk of contamination and infection due to repeated punctures, frequent connections and manipulations. Skin germs have a special affinity to plastics. Colonisation occurs on the inner and outer surface producing a biofilm with staphylococcal coagulase. The metabolism and catabolites of these germs may contribute to chronic inflammatory processes, to flow obstructions by thrombogenesis and fibrino-genesis and provoke infection or sepsis.

7.1.6.1 Handling Prosthetic Shunts

Compared to AV shunts higher requirements have to be respected during the needle placement, connection and compression.

- Sterile gloves, masks and sterile sheet to prepare the puncture materials needed for shall be used.
- The patient shall wear a protective mask or turn away the face during the needle placement and shall not speak.
- The puncture sites must be covered with sterile dressing during treatment as well as after removal of the needles.

- The compression must be performed with sterile compresses.
- Alternatively, sterile gloves must be used for direct compression of the puncture site.

7.1.6.2 Handling Central Venous Catheters and Port Systems

Catheter-related bacteraemia is one of the most frequent cause of catheter failure. Double-lumen catheters are apparently more affected than single-lumen catheters.

Remark:
The frequent connections as well as the single flow direction in double lumen catheters (arterial and venous side) can be reasons for a significantly high colonisation of lumen.[83]

The connection and disconnection of temporary CVCs and implanted atrial catheters and port systems must be carried out under the same protective hygienic measures as described for prosthetic shunts. A sterile sheet must be used within the immediate area of the catheter or port. A second sheet can be used to prepare the sterile material.

The high number of manipulations on catheter connections and port systems shall be reduced to a minimum using standardised working techniques.

The use of SN adapters in single-lumen catheters or additional catheter extension pieces in double-lumen catheters can reduce the number of direct connections at the catheter connectors and increase the hygienic standard[84].

---

[83] RKI-Empfehlung: Prävention Gefäßkatheter-assoziierter Infektionen. Bundesgesundheitsbl. – Gesundheitsforsch – Gesundheitsschutz 2002 (45): 907-924 (www.rki.de)

[84] Gorke, A.: Mikrobiologische Kontamination von Hämodialyse-Katheter-Anschlüssen. Journal für das Nephrologische Team, 2003 (2): 88-93

7.1.6.3 Care of the Catheter Exit Site (CES)

The inspection of the CES must and the change of dressing/care of the CES can be done before the connection. The final dressing can also be put on after the treatment.
The CES classification can be derived from Twadorsky's PD classification[85].

Classification of CES of CVCs	Evaluation	Measures
Perfect CES	no inflammatory signs intact skin vicinity	
Threatening CES infections		
a) irritated CES	dry crust without reddening	
b) Infection-threatened CES	superficial, dry to moderate cutaneous lesion (< 0.25 cm)	Swab test, systematic antibiosis if necessary
Acute CES infection	Reddening > 0.25 cm Crusts, purulent or blood exudate	Smear test: germ identification mandatory systemic antibiosis
Chronic CES infection	Reddening, crusts, exudate, longer than 4 weeks	Smear test: systemic antibiosis, catheter explantation if necessary
Tunnel infection	Infection exceeds outer muffle in direction towards the heart	sonography-diagnosis catheter explantation systemic antibiosis

Air turbulence , e.g. caused by open windows and doors and unnecessary movements, shall be avoided during the care of CES as well as during the connection and disconnection phases.

[85] Twardowsky, Z.J.: Current approach to exit-site infections in patients on peritoneal dialysis. Nephrol Dial Transplant 1997 (12): 1284

For the care of CES, CVC and port only sterile materials and aseptic working techniques must be used. Non-sterile dressings do not comply with the requirement and shall not be used. They could only be used for the peripheral and external fixation of the catheter.

There are not many publications on dressing materials like polyurethane, hydrocolloid, hydropolymer and polyacrylamide dressings for CVC from the field of dialysis.

The type of CES dressing e.g. transparent or occlusive, determines whether the dressing has to be changed at each treatment session. Highly permeable dressings from e.g. polyurethane material can be left on for up to 7 days. Transparent dressing must have a moisture permeability of at least 500 ml/m/24 hrs/37 °C. Transparent dressings shall only be used on non-irritated and perfect exits[86].

Taking a shower can be recommended for patients with non-irritated or perfect CES. The catheter and its dressing will be covered with a waterproof plastic dressing foil; the dressing will be changed afterwards.

Patients with infected CES or in the postoperative phase shall not be allowed to shower.

If the dressing is soaked or contaminated or if there is suspicion of an infection, the dressing must be changed immediately.

In case of irritation or surface infection of the CES, the dressing has to be changed at each hemodialysis session. Smear testing is mandatory for irritated and infected CES.

[86] Mermel, L.A.: Prevention of Intravascular Catheter Related Infection. Annals of Internal Medicine, 2000 (132 (5)): 7

Summary of dressings:

Material	Properties	Safety	Rationale	Change
Polyester film ("wallpaper dressing"), sterile, non-sterile	adheres well, permeable to humidity, contaminated when stored openly	No	Aggressive adhesive, plaster allergies, painful during removal, skin lesions probable, permeable to humidity in both directions	every treatment session
Highly permeable, transparent dressings, sterile	sealed to humidity from outside, permeable from inside	Yes	Only in non-irritable CES; eudermic; optimal optical evaluation; reduced frequency and workload for change	up to 7 days
Sterile wound/ bed plaster	resorbing effect	Yes	for non-irritated, irritated or infected CES	every 2nd day

Medications administered (for CES-treatment) shall be specific and their application shall follow planned/prescribed intervals. Ointments shall only be applied during dialysis and removed at the end of the dialysis session. According to findings a dry sterile dressing is attached after each dialysis session or more frequently.

Remark:
The prophylactic application of antibiotic ointments and solvents is still reported but does not have a proven effect; it can lead to skin irritation and microbiological resistance. Ointments are only effective within a defined period of time and can later promote the growth of germs.

7.1.6.4 Cleaning Agents and Disinfectants for the CES

Non-irritated CES can be cleaned with sterile physiological sodium chloride solution or aseptic disinfectant solutions using sterile compresses.

Approved disinfectants and procedures have to be used in disinfecting the skin around the CES. Due to the possibility of interactions with materials, disinfectants shall be released for use by the manufacturer of the catheter or the ports. Substances like wound petroleum ether and acetone partially used for cleaning are damaging the skin through dehydration. Hydrogen peroxide is cytotoxic in the CES area[87, 88]. Alcohol-containing disinfectants have a short exposure time for skin disinfection; they are however not advisable for irritated CES. The manufacturer needs to be contacted for information about possible interaction with the catheter materials.

Polyvidon iodine-containing disinfectants are not recommended because of the long exposure time (up to 5 minutes) and skin coloration which is limiting assessment of the site. The risk of a iodine allergy and wound healing disturbances as well as the interaction with other disinfectants are described.

Other disinfectants or antiseptic agents like Polyhexanide and Octenidine have an acceptable exposure time and demonstrate good skin tolerance and effectiveness especially on irritated and infected CES. For information on possible interactions with catheter materials the manufacturer shall be contacted.

7.1.6.5 Cleaning Agents and Disinfectants for the Catheter Connectors

Ideally, the same disinfectant shall be used for disinfection of the catheter connectors and CES. The status of the CES and characteristics of access material must be considered when choosing the disinfectants and disinfection procedures.

[87] Kusel, C.: Wundbehandlung – zeitgemäß – professionell – effektiv. Pflegen Ambulant, 12. Jahrg. 2001 (4): 26-29

[88] Kramer, A. et al.: Konsensusempfehlung zur Auswahl von Wirkstoffen für die Wundantiseptik. ZfW 2004 (3): 110-120

Substances like wound petroleum ether, acetone, sodium hypochlorite and hydrogen peroxide shall not be used when cleaning the catheter connections.

The manufacturer shall be contacted for information on interaction with catheter material when using alcoholic disinfectants. Polyvidon iodine-containing disinfectants are not to be recommended due to the long exposure time (up to 5 minutes) and adhesions and coloured alterations.

The manufacturer shall be contacted for information about possible interaction of other disinfectants like Polyhexanide and Octenidine with catheter material.

Remark:
The target is a reduction of the number of manipulations at the catheter hubs. SN adapters or catheter extensions used in double-lumen catheters shall be connected dry immediately after the disinfection of the catheter connections and removal of the connector cap. All further manipulations like taking blood, internal rinsing through the catheter hubs with saline, etc. shall be performed at the distal connection sites of the extension. "Non-Touch technique" and sterile materials have to be used without any further disinfection or cleaning at the extension site.

7.1.6.6 Lock Solutions for CES and Port Systems

Sterile lock solutions shall keep the lumen of the catheter or port system open; they shall not provoke any material deterioration and put the patient at risk. The lock-solution shall not provoke microbial growth and biofilm formation[89, 90].

The quantity of lock solution depends on the length of the catheter and the lumen. The use of vials that have been opened and used before is not allowed for reasons of sterility.

[89] Polaschegg, H.D., Sodemann, K.: Der DIALOCK Blutzugangsport kombiniert mit einer antimikrobiellen Lock-Lösung verbessert die Lebensdauer, Sicherheit und Folgekosten von Kathetern. EDTNA/ERCA Journal XXVIII, 2002 (1): 31-36

[90] Weijmer, M.C. et al.: Superior Antimicrobial Activity of Trisodium Citrate Over Heparin for Catheter Locking., NDT, 2002 (17): 2164-2169

The application shall be performed slowly and only after sufficient rinsing with saline due to laminar flow effects.

Up to now, catheter manufacturers recommend the application of standard Heparin. Other substances like e.g. Tri-Sodium-Citrate (TSC) in different concentrations with and without supplements are also in use. Compared to standard Heparin, citrate solutions of high and low concentrations act bacteria-static to certain microbes e.g. skin bacteria.

The use of a number of alternative lock solutions has been reported in the literature, e.g. Vitamin C, isotonic or high concentrated sodium chloride solution, diluted Heparin solution, Lepirudin, Danaparoid or fibrinolytic agents. Valid studies have still to be carried out.

In case of heparin-induced thrombocytopenia (HIT II), the catheter has to be locked with a heparin-free solution.

7.1.6.7 Microbiological Analysis

Prior to antibiotic treatment, swab testing from locally irritated and potentially infected puncture sites as well as the CES have to be carried with sterile cotton wool swabs soaked in NaCl 0.9%.

In case of a suspicion or evidence of catheter related infection or sepsis, a blood culture from the catheter lumen and from a peripheral vein must be taken prior to antibiotic treatment. The ratio of the microbes found in the different samples can provide information about the source of the infection.

After removing the catheter, the tip of the catheter may be sent to a laboratory with appropriate experience in testing samples of catheter material. The values of the findings are given in cfu/ml with and without differentiation.

7.1.7 Home Dialysis – Aspects of Vascular Access

Home dialysis patients (home haemodialysis, peritoneal dialysis) shall be instructed and educated, and regularly re-educated by specialised nephrology nurses. The special content includes aspects of vascular access hygiene:

- safe aseptic handling during needle setting and exit dressing
- evaluation of vascular access and its function, long-term evaluation
- handling sterile material
- adequate action in case of problems with vascular and peritoneal access.

7.2 Home Dialysis Treatment

7.2.1 Goal and Rationale

In home dialysis treatment, the protection and safety of the patient and his domestic help (if necessary) shall be a top priority. Structured and documented home dialysis education shall support the patient and home dialysis partner to independently carry out the treatment and identify and avoid dangerous situations regarding hygiene in time.

A well-educated and experienced treatment team must be available at all times for consultation and assistance in decision-making. In home treatment there is no risk of cross-contamination. The hygienic requirements can differ from those of Out-patient and In-patient treatment facilities. Goals, individual and practically-orientated solutions shall be sought jointly.

7.2.2 Home Haemodialysis

There is no relevant difference regarding the technical equipment and the realisation of the dialysis in home haemodialysis and centre or hospital-based dialysis. All basic rules apply for the prevention of infections, regarding water purification, connecting vascular access, haemodialysis fluids, maintenance of dialysis machines, use of sterile materials and waste disposal apply. The difference is in the home ambience and the legal responsibility for the treatment. Within the framework of home dialysis for example, the patient is a self-care person and also considered the "operator" in regard to the Medical Device Act (MPG) and the Drinking Water Ordinance (TWV).

The requirements for the preconditions on the building, installations, water purification, treatment area and the running operations are tabled in the check list "Requirements to Home Dialysis" (s. ch. 11.1).

7.2.3 Peritoneal Dialysis (PD)

The therapeutical success of the procedure essentially depends on the long-term avoidance of peritonitis and its consequences for the peritoneum. The hygienic risks include mainly manipulations on the PD catheter and the catheter exit. The evaluation of infection signs is an important part of the education[91]. Peritoneal dialysis can normally be carried out by the patient alone without a treatment partner.

The requirements concerning the structural preconditions, the treatment area and the running operation are shown in tabular form in the check list "Peritoneal Dialysis – Preconditions and Operation" in ch. 11.2.

---

[91] De Vijt, D. et al.: Post Insertion Catheter Care in Peritoneal Dialysis Centres across Europe. EDTNA/ERCA Journal, XXX, 2004 (2): 101-106

7.2.3.1 Requirements for Catheter Implantation

The overall aim is a good acceptance of the catheter by the body of the patient, the avoidance of long-term consequences such as peritonitis and CES and tunnel infections and the maintenance of a non-irritable catheter exit site (CES).The PD catheter, e.g. Tenkhoff, Oreopoulos-Zellermann catheters, must be placed under aseptic conditions. The procedures following the operation standard show the best result.

In catheter care four different stages shall be considered:
- care in the phase before catheter implantation
- care immediately after the implantation
- care in a non-irritated or perfect exit site
- care in case of inflamed catheter exit site

7.2.3.2 Nursing Care for Preparing Catheter Implantation

Special preparatory measures e.g. complete purgation, treatment of nasal Staphylococcus aureus diagnosis, planning the CES and informing the patient about post-operative behaviour like bed rest for example can increase the success of creating a non-irritating, complication-free catheter system.

7.2.3.3 Nursing Care Immediately after the Implantation

A sterile dressing shall be attached on the exit-site in the operation room, the initial dressing shall be left for 2 to 3 days without being renewed if possible. The catheter exit site is covered with sterile compresses, and the catheter is secured pressure-free and tension-free. The fixation is done with sterile dressing material. It is necessary to check the dressing daily. Blood soaked or wet dressings must be changed immediately.

7.2.3.4 Nursing Care in Non-Irritable or Perfect Exit Site

The change of dressing during the postoperative phase (ca. 10 days) has to be carried out with sterile gloves as well as mouth/ nasal protection. The examination and changing of the dressing must be carried out by an experienced nephrological specialist nurse or by a physician having experience with the procedure.

The patient has to be educated by the experienced specialist nurse. At home he changes the dressing daily and identifies alterations in time. A perfect and good CES develops epithelisation and requires no dressing. Securing the catheter extension is however necessary in order to keep any pressure or traction away from the catheter. Infection prevention is achieved by daily inspection of CES and appropriate personal hygiene.

7.2.3.5 Nursing Care of the Inflamed Catheter Exit Site

According to Twardowsky[92] a total of 5 different manifestations of a CES infection can be differentiated (ch. 7.1.6.3).

An infection of the CES appears with reddening, swelling and purulent secretion.

Pathogens in the secretion shall be laboratory confirmed with a swab.

The cleaning and disinfection of the exit site and the changing of the dressing have to be done on a daily basis and under the same aseptic conditions like in the postoperative changing of dressing.

The cleaning or disinfecting solution must be sterile. They shall be manufactured and packed in small containers, shall have no toxic side-effects and be non-irritant to the skin.

[92] Twardowsky, Z. J. et al.: Current approach to exit-site infections in patients on peritoneal dialysis. Nephrol. Dial. Transplant., 1997 (12): 1284

Pharmacological treatment shall be done systemically and locally with an appropriate antibiotic according to the results of the antibiotic resistance test[93]. Administration of antibiotics shall be determined by a antibiotic resistance test and carried out by an experienced nurse or the patient himself at home. The duration of antibiotic treatment shall be determined by the physician, based on the course of the infection. The transition system shall be changed under sterile conditions.

For further clarification an ultrasonic examination of the catheter's course (discrimination of CES or tunnel infection) as well as a nasal swab and if necessary further clarification of cause and further education of the patient shall take place.

In case of nasal colonisation with Staphylococcus aureus an antibiotic therapy using Mupirocin ointment for example can be carried out.

7.2.3.6 Dressing Material

When selecting plastic foil dressings, it has to be regarded that these have a steam permeability rate of at least 500 ml/m/24 hrs/ 37 °C. Plastic foil dressings shall be applied only on non-irritated and perfect exits.

7.2.3.7 Shower

Showers could be recommended to patients with non-irritated or perfect exit sites. The catheter extension has to be secured during the shower and no traction shall be exercised on the catheter. Patients with inflamed CES or in the postoperative phase shall not be allowed to shower.

[93] Keane, W.F. et al.: Adult peritoneal dialysis-related treatment recommendations 2000 update. Perit. Dial. Int., 2000 (20): 396

7.2.3.8 Bath

The patient can bath and swim in saline-containing or relatively cold waters (sea or lake). It is not documented whether a waterproof film can minimise bacterial infection. Bathing can only be recommended to patients with non-irritated or perfect CES.

7.2.3.9 Changing the Transfer Set

The catheter transfer set has to be changed according to the instructions of the manufacturer under aseptic conditions and with a filled peritoneal cavity by an experienced PD specialist nurse. After that, the bag has to be changed and the dialysate drained before the next inflow. A hygienic disinfection of the hands must be carried out, sterile gloves and surgical mask must be worn.

7.2.3.10 Exchanging the Dialysis Solutions

The dialysis solution must be exchanged under aseptic conditions. Here, a surgical mask must be worn and the hands shall be thoroughly disinfected respecting the exposure time of 30 seconds. Washing the hands before disinfection is necessary only in case of serious contamination. Jewellery (watches, chains, rings) have to be removed before disinfecting the hands.

7.2.3.11 Supplements to the Dialysis Solution

The injection of pharmacological products e.g. insulin or antibiotics into the dialysis solution must be carried out under aseptic conditions and shall be reduced to a minimum. The wearing of a surgical mask as well as a thorough disinfection of the hands is mandatory.

7.3 Special Epidemiological Aspects

7.3.1 Goal and Rationale

Avoidance of contamination and cross-contamination with transmissible pathogens in dialysis by following consistent hygienic procedures must be aimed for. For the possible blood-transmittable viral infections there is an increased risk for the development of a chronic course of infection with a resulting negative influence on the prognosis of the patient. In all infectious diseases the special out-patient treatment situation, the additional psychological stress due to quarantine measures, the special requirements on the organisation and the additional resulting costs shall be considered.

7.3.2 Blood-Transmissible Viral Infections (Hep. B, Hep. C, HIV and Others)

7.3.2.1 General

Haemodialysis-associated infections are considered to be those which are transmitted more frequently under haemodialysis conditions. The most important among these viral infections are the frequently parenteral transmitted hepatitis B and hepatitis C infections. For other parenteral infections transmitted through blood like e.g. the HGV-C- ("hepatitis G") or the TT-virus infection (transfusion-transmitted virus), it is likewise not seldom that chronic virus carriers present high viral loads in the blood, but no pathogenic signs could be proven so far.

Out of about 58,000 dialysis patients in Germany, 2003 were infectious patients[94] out of which

- 571 were Hepatitis B positive
- 1662 Hepatitis C positive
- 51 HIV positive

[94] Quasi-Niere: Nierenersatztherapie in Deutschland. Bericht über Dialysebehandlung und Nierentransplantation in Deutschland 2003a, 2004 (www.quasi-niere.de)

The prevention of transmission of blood-transmissible infections depends mainly on the strict adherence of the hygienic measures. During invasive activities on the patient, the staff shall not take care of any other patients even in cases of emergency. Organisational regulations have to be defined in the hygiene plan.

Transfusion of blood or blood products can also be the source of infection for new HBV and HCV infections. With an HBV and HCV carrier rate of 0.5 to 1% within the German population in the past, transfusions of blood and especially those from pooled non-inactivated blood products, e.g. preparations of coagulation factors, have caused a very high risk of infection. Various studies demonstrated that in the past, the transfusion of blood was also a risk factor for dialysis patients especially for HCV infections.

Transmission of infections from infected patients to staff is often caused by needle-stick injuries. There is an HBV transmission rate of 10-20% after inoculation of the HBsAg-positive blood, about 3% transmission rate with anti-HCV-positive blood and a rate of 0.32% with anti-HIV-positive blood[95].

7.3.2.2 Information and Education about Viral Infections Transmitted via Blood

Patients with confirmed HBV, HCV, and HIV infections must be informed about the prognosis of their illness, the therapeutic possibilities and about the risk to infect others such as family members, fellow patients, medical staff or when donating blood. They shall be sent to an internal consultant as early as possible so that further examinations necessary for establishing the prognosis and therapy can be carried out, e.g. liver puncture, viral load determination, HCV genotype determination, CD4 cell count in case of HIV infection and so that the optimal point of time for the onset of

[95] Aktualisierte Empfehlungen 2002 zur beruflichen Exposition mit Blut und biologischen Flüssigkeiten, Fachkomission Klinik und Therapie HIV/AIDS des Bundesamtes für Gesundheit, Bulletin 10: 192-196 und Fragebögen

therapy is not missed, e.g. interferon treatment of Hepatitis B and C before a kidney transplantation, antiviral chemotherapy of the HIV infection on attaining a critical CD4 cell count.

7.3.2.3 Prevention of Transmission of Infections

In case of new occurrence of hepatitis infections in the dialysis unit, the source of infection and the most likely mode of transmission shall be found. This will help to prevent further infections. At the same time, sources of infection outside the dialysis unit like holiday dialysis, the transfusion of blood and blood products, persons with hepatitis in the flat-sharing community or with intimate partners and intravenous drug consumption shall be looked for and ruled out.

If there is a transmission within the dialysis unit, this happens mostly indirectly from patient to patient through contaminated hands and surfaces. If HBV and HCV infections break out among dialysis patients, dialysis staff who are chronically infected with these viruses shall be ruled out as a source of infection.

A commonly used means of identifying the source of infection is the sequencing of a part of the virus genome that shows high variability.

If the source of infection has been located, information about the mode of transmission can be collected by analysing the possibilities of contact between the source of infection and the newly infected patients (for example, dialysis on an adjacent machine during the same dialysis shift, use of the same machine during another shift, "sharing" the same nurse/person of staff) and due to the chronology of the infection. This is important to identify the weak points in infection prevention and to avoid further infections.

Machines and Rooms

For patients with blood-transmittable viral infections, separate dialysis machines shall be used[96]. These machines are to be marked in a way that they can be assigned to the respective group of infected patients.

Dialysis machines which have been used for infected patients may be reused in non-infectious sections only after carrying out corresponding procedures. The precondition is the documented reprocessing of the machines according to details described in ch. 6.5.3.

HBV, HCV and HIV infected patients shall be dialysed while separated spatially and if necessary temporarily from non-infectious patients as well as from patients with another infection.

Remark:
The treatment room can for example be used as follows:
1st shift: non-infectious patients; 2nd shift: infectious patients. In such a changing occupancy of rooms it has to be observed that between the two shifts, all surfaces near to the patients, all work surfaces, the hand basin (including the fittings) as well as all the surfaces which come into contact with the skin are disinfected with approved agents and procedures which are effective against viruses.

Disposal of Infectious Needles

The filler opening of the container for disposal of used needles can be a source for contamination and infections. Separate bins for disposal of used needles and waste containers shall be used for the individual infectious groups. Changing the disposable gloves immediately after disposing the needles can be necessary.

[96] Anlagen zur Richtlinie für Krankenhaushygiene und Infektionsprävention (www.rki.de)

Staff Safety[97]

The status of staff of a dialysis unit regarding infection with HBV and HCV and after special consent for HIV has to be recorded.

Remark:
HIV testing does not arise from the Biological Agents Ordinance.

Staff shall be vaccinated against hepatitis B.

Surgical mask and safety glasses or a complete face protection mask shall be worn for all interventions during which a risk of splash of blood is given or possible contact with other body fluids. Staff wear clean work clothes which have to be changed daily. If direct contact with blood or contaminated objects is to be expected, then disposable gloves and protective overalls or fluid-repelling aprons shall be worn additionally over the work clothes. The additional overalls or aprons are to be used depending on the section, e.g. infectious section. The overall shall be replaced immediately if there is any visible contamination or soiling.

The measures to be undertaken in case of needle injury or eye contact with infectious blood shall be defined in the hygiene plan. Newly contaminated or infected staff have to present themselves to the authorised medical insurance examiner. A conservative and if described drug supported post exposure prophylaxis (PEP) has to be carried out.

Visitors

Visitors, craftsmen, technicians and consultants have to be made aware of the possible risks of infection. Protective overalls and hygienic disinfection of the hands can be necessary.

[97] BioStoffV

Linen

Linen from patients with viral infections has to be changed as described in ch. 6.2.7 and in ch. 11.12.

Linen contaminated with pathogens of the so called "notifiable diseases" according to the Infections Protection Act has to be specially registered and labelled[98].

7.3.2.4 Immunisation (vaccination) for Dialysis Patients and Staff

Due to the reduced immune reaction of dialysis patients, the course of infections can be especially fulminated. Due to this there is an urgent indication for immunisation against other vaccine-preventable infections in addition to the immunisation against hepatitis B. The attained antibody titres and the persistence of the antibodies usually is less than the values found in those who are immunocompetent[99].

An influenza vaccination shall be done every year in autumn using the latest influenza vaccine available. Due to their underlying disease, dialysis patients are especially endangered to develop difficult and partially deadly complications (especially primary influenza pneumonia and secondary bacterial pneumonia). All medical staff shall also have yearly vaccination. Vaccination of the staff is not only for their personal protection but also for the safety and protection of the patients most at risk for infections transmitted by staff. The routine influenza vaccination can reduce the number of sick employees thereby saving costs for the employer. A vaccination with an unconjugated pneumococcus-polysaccharide vaccine is recommended every 3-5 years according to the US

---

[98] BGR 250/TRBA 250, ch. 7.2

[99] CDC: Recommendations for Preventing Transmission of Infections among Chronic Haemodialysis Patients. MMWR, 2001 (50, N° RR-5)

Advisory Committee on Immunisation Practices[100]. Toxoid vaccines against tetanus and diphtheria shall be given in the same doses (children aged 5 years and over with a reduced dose of diphtheria vaccine) and within the same interval (booster injection every 10 years) as in healthy persons. At present there is a clinical study conducted in the U.S. on a vaccine against Staphylococcus aureus which shall finish in 2006.[101]

7.3.3 Hepatitis B

In the history of dialysis, there have been repeated HBV epidemics in which a high rate of contamination of patients and staff have been observed in dialysis centres[102]. In 1990, the average carrier rate of HBsAg in European dialysis patients was still 6.1%. However, there were strong regional differences.

The introduction of strict hygienic measures combined with the regular immunisation of patients and staff against hepatitis B since 1982 has, however, led to a considerable decline in the rate of infection (at present the infection rate in the U.S.A. is just about 0.1% p.a.) and of the HBsAg carrier rate.

7.3.3.1 Route of Infection and Risk Factors of HBV Infection

HBV is a relatively stable DNA virus which is found in high concentrations in the blood. Just a ten millionth part of a millilitre can transfer the infection. The virus remains active for days in dried blood on contaminated surfaces and instruments. Due to this,

[100] Prevention of Pneumococcal Diseases: Recommendations of the Advisory Committee on Immunisation Practices (ACIP). Morb. Mortal. Wkly Rep., 1997 (46): 1-24

[101] Shinfield H. et al.: Use of a Staphylococcus aureus Conjugate Vaccine in Patients Receiving Haemodialysis. New England Journal of Medicine, 2002 (346): 491-496 (http://content.nejm.org)

[102] EDTA/ERA Registry Reports, 1972-1994

there is a danger of indirect transmission of the virus from patient to patient through the smallest amounts of blood invisible to the eye which can be found on jointly used devices, e.g. sphygmomanometers, in jointly used injection solutions, e.g. heparin, or on the gloves of dialysis staff and from there, they find their way into the bloodstream or onto the mucosa of predisposed persons.

This transfer of infectious blood is facilitated when HBsAg carriers are dialysed without any spatial separations to predisposed persons and the same staff takes care of HBV infected patients as well as patients who are not immune against hepatitis B[103, 104].

7.3.3.2 HBV-Diagnostics in Dialysis Patients

After referral of new patients to the dialysis unit there shall be immediate testing for possible infection of HBV and immune status. A test for HBsAg, anti-HBc, and anti-HBs is carried out. If an HBsAg test is positive, it has to be confirmed mostly with the help of a neutralisation test, because false positive results are possible. Until clarification of the infection status, the patient shall be treated with his own dialysis machine. For confirmed positive tests, the patient is sent to the group of patients infected with HBV.

If only the anti-HBc test is positive, i.e. no HBsAg or a virus can be detected by means of the PCR at the same time, this indicates that there has been a previous contact with the HBV.

There are four possibilities available with so-called "anti-HBc only patients" in the serological routine panel (in which the viral DNA proof with PCR is not included):

[103] CDC: Recommendations for Preventing Transmission of Infections among Chronic Haemodialysis Patients. MMWR, 2001 (50, N° RR-5)

[104] Froio N. et al.: Contamination by Hepatitis B and C Viruses in the Dialysis Setting. Am J Kidney Dis 2003 (42): 546-550

- He has just got over an acute HBV infection
- He is immune after an infection, but still has a very low anti-HBs serum level which is not detectable in the routine tests.
- The anti-HBc proof is falsely positive
- He has a chronic HBV infection with a very low, non-detectable HBs-AG serum concentration. The last is the case in at least 30% of the patients, but then the HBV-DNA detection is positive with PCR.

Testing for HBV-DNA using the PCR shall always be carried out on patients showing isolated anti-HBc-positive results. If the HBV-DNA is detectable, the patient is infectious and shall be isolated.

If the HBV-DNA is not detectable, the patient shall be vaccinated. A previous infection can also be confirmed if after a single hepatitis B vaccination there is an anti-HBs concentration of more than 100 IU/l during evaluation of the immunisation response. If this is not the case, a complete primary basic immunisation against hepatitis B shall be carried out[105].

It is sufficient to evaluate HBsAg and anti-HBc during the semi-annual or additional checks for HBV infections. Shall anti-HBc and/or HBsAg be positive for the first time, testing for anti-HBc IgM has to be carried out. Its presence is proof of a fresh HBV infection. It is to be noted that the HBsAg test can still be positive for almost two weeks after the hepatitis B vaccination without confirmation of an HBV infection. Thus no test to check the HBsAg shall be carried out during the vaccination phase in order to avoid false results.

As an additional indication of hepatitis infections, the transaminase value of the GOT and GPT shall be checked in monthly or quarterly intervals.

[105] Reichen J., P.J. Grob im Namen der SEVHEP (Schweizer Experten für Virale Hepatitis): Hepatitis B Virusinfektion: Diagnose, klinische Folgen, Therapie und Prophylaxe. Praxis 2002 (91): 307-319 (http://www.systoc.com/outcomes_protocols/hepatitisB_Panel.htm)

Remark:
Sensitivity and specificity of the transaminase value in HBV and HCV diagnostics: The sensitivity of this examination is not optimal especially during a chronic infection. In a considerable part of chronic HBV and HCV infections, no increase of the transaminase value is seen. However, in about 80% of the cases a fresh HBV infection leads to an increase in the values which are already present 1-2 months before the occurrence of anti-HCV and almost simultaneous with the occurrence of HCV-RNA[106].
Due to the fact that non-infected dialysis patients on average present lower transaminase values as normal persons[107], already a relatively small increase of the values above the level of previous tests gives reason for the serological clarification of an HBV or HCV infection (s. ch. 11.6. HBV Diagnosis and ch. 11.7. HCV Diagnosis).
Increased transaminase values can also be due to other causes, e.g. alcohol, medicine, physical exertion, hyperhydration with hepatic congestion and other viral diseases involving the liver, e.g. Coxsackie-Virus, Epstein-Barr-Virus. They do not prove the presence of a viral hepatitis.

7.3.3.3 HBV Exposure of Staff or Patients

In general, every exposure shall be documented.

A confirmed infection of the staff has to be reported as an occupational illness. After a probable exposure of the staff or patients to the HBV, e.g. through a needle-prick inoculation from the blood of someone infected with HBV, blood contact with mucosa, eyes or wounds, it is necessary to carry out the post exposure prophylaxis recommended by the Permanent Vaccination Commission (STIKO) following the interval and the success of previous hepatitis B vaccinations (s. ch. 11.10 HBV Post Exposure Prophylaxis)[108].

---

[106] Saab S. et al.: Serum alanine aminotransferase in hepatitis C screening of patients on haemodialysis. Am. J. Kidney Dis., 2001 (37): 308-315

[107] Espinosa M. et al.: High ALT levels predict viremia in anti-HCV-positive HD patients if a modified normal range of ALT is applied. Clin. Nephrol., 2000 (54): 151-156

[108] Sarrazin U., Brodt H., Sarrazin C., Zeuzem S.: Prophylaxe gegenüber HBV, HCV und HIV nach beruflicher Exposition, Dtsch Ärztebl 2005 (102): A 2234-2239

No measures are necessary for staff if the primary immunisation (anti-HBs > 100 IU/l) is less than 5 years back or if an anti-HBs concentration of > 100 IU/l was measured within the last 12 months. It is recommended to give one single booster dose of the vaccine if immunisation was successfully carried out within the last 5-10 years. In other cases, e.g. if the immunisation was not complete or if not performed at all, if the success of the vaccination was never checked, if the person is a low responder after vaccination, if the immunisation is more than 10 years old, an immediate quantitative antibody test will decide on how to proceed further: with more than 100 IU/l no measures will be taken; with 10-100 IU/l just a booster injection has to be administered; with less than 10 IU/l or if there is the impossibility of testing within 48 hours, then an immediate passive-active immunisation has to be carried out while at the same time hepatitis B immuno-globulin has to be administered and the hepatitis B immunisation has to be initiated or completed.

After the end of the incubation period of maximum 6 months, the success of the post exposure prophylaxis has to be checked: HBsAg and anti-HBc have to remain negative. In so far as hepatitis B immuno-globulin has also been administered, the incubation period can be more than 9 months and the testing has to be repeated after 12 months. Without post exposure prophylaxis, a transmission rate of 10-20% has to be expected after needle-stick injury with HBsAg-positive blood.

If patients are exposed to the HBV, no measures are to be introduced if after successful primary immunisation within the last 12 months an anti-HBs value of > 100 IU/l was measured. In all other cases, the antibody level shall be determined immediately and a post exposure prophylaxis as described earlier shall be initiated. Due to the insufficient immune response of the chronic dialysis patient the doses of preparations and vaccines as well as the frequency of the measures have to be increased.

7.3.3.4 Hepatitis B Immunisation of Staff and Patients

In case of hepatitis B, there is the possibility of a immuno-prophylaxis by immunisation (active immunisation) and the administration of hepatitis B immuno-globulin (passive immunisation).

Patients and staff shall be vaccinated against hepatitis B. The dosage scheme is comprised of 3 or 4 vaccinations in intervals of 0, 1 and 6 months or 0, 1, 2 and 6 months. Using these schedules it has to be noted that a basic immunisation interrupted throughout years has to be completed only by the remaining number of vaccine doses. Quotation of the Permanent Vaccination Commission (STIKO): "There are no inadmissible intervals between vaccinations. Every vaccination counts. Even a primary immunisation that was interrupted for many years must not be completely repeated!"[109]

According to STIKO, the success of an immunisation has to be checked via means of an anti-HBs test 4 weeks after the vaccination. An immunisation is considered successful if an anti-HBs-concentration of at least 100 IU/l is reached. If the concentration is between 10 and 100 IU/l ("low responder"), an additional dose of vaccine followed by evaluation of response shall be administered. If less than 100 IU/l are still measured or after 3 vaccinations or anti-HBs is still not detectable (< 10 IU/l; "non-responder"), then a second vaccination cycle shall be completed or carried out (i.e. the administration of a total of 6 vaccine doses).

About 5% of the staff and up to 50% of the dialysis patients do not develop anti-HBs after regular immunisation and are probably not protected from hepatitis B. Through the above-mentioned second immunisation cycle, a sufficient formation of antibodies can still be initiated in about half of the number of low and non-responders.

[109] Empfehlungen der Ständigen Impfkommission (STIKO) am Robert-Koch-Institut, Stand: Juli 2004. Epidemiologisches Bulletin 23. Juli 2004 (30): 235-250

The success of the immunisation on dialysis patients increases when administering a double dose of the vaccine[110, 111].

When the patients are vaccinated earlier, possibly before the beginning of the dialysis treatment, the rate of non-responders appears to be clearly lower.

According to the recommendations of the STIKO, dialysis staff as well as patients with persisting antibody level shall receive a booster injection 10 years after the basic vaccination.

For patients with a titre below 50 IU/l (s. ch. 11.6 HBV Diagnosis) during the 6 months of control, a booster injection with the double dose shall be carried out immediately.

Remark:
Due to a rapid decline of antibodies and a possibly shorter duration of the immunity of dialysis patients, the European Dialysis and Transplant Association recommends the testing of quantitative anti-HBs every 6 months and the administration of a booster injection when the anti-HBs concentration falls below 10 IU/l[112].

Compared to subcutaneous applications, the intradermal application of the vaccine on dialysis patients is equivalent to the intramuscular application with regards to success and tolerance of the immunisation[113].

---

[110] CDC: Recommendations for Preventing Transmission of Infections among Chronic Haemodialysis Patients. MMWR, 2001 (50, N° RR-5)

[111] O.M.G.E. Organisation Mondiale de Gastro-Entérologie (www.omge.org/guidelines)

[112] European Renal Association – European Dialysis and Transplant Association. Section IV. Haemodialysis-associated infections. Nephrol. Dial. Tansplant. 2002 (17 (Suppl. 7)): 72-87

[113] Charest A. F. et al.: A randomised comparison of intradermal and intramuscular vaccination against hepatitis B virus in incident chronic haemodialysis patients. Am. J. Kidney Dis., 2000 (36 (5)): 976-982

7.3.4 Hepatitis C

Nowadays Hep C is the dominant form of hepatitis virus in dialysis units, still no immuno-prophylaxis in form of an immunisation or immunglobulin dose exists. In the past years, the nosocomial transmission mostly from patients to patients could be confirmed in a large number of epidemics with the help of molecular virological methods.

In 1995, a total of 14.4% of the patients and 2.0% of the staff in 2647 dialysis centres in the USA with 224954 patients and 54194 staff were positive for antibodies against hepatitis C (Anti-HCV)[114]. Until 2000, the contamination has fallen from 8.4% to 1.6% due to hygienic measures applied. In a study published in 2002, 2796 patients in 43 dialysis centres in Germany were observed, 7% of the patients were found to have an existing or subsided HCV infection out of which 4% had viremia (HCV-RNA positive)[115].

7.3.4.1 Routes of Infection and Risk Factors of HCV Infection

HCV is less stable than HBV. Therefore, transmission through blood-contaminated devices does not appear to take place so easily. At present, however, there is no consent whether the strict observance of hygienic measures alone is sufficient to prevent the transmission of the infection as is apparently the case with HIV. It could however be shown in various studies that the treatment of patients in large dialysis units represented an unfavourable ratio of patients to staff and the treatment of "white" patients in the same shift or adjacent to an HCV infected patient represent risk factors which can not be neglected.

[114] Tokars J.I. et al.: National surveillance of dialysis associated diseases in the United States, 1995. ASAIO J., 1998 Jan-Feb (44 (1)): 98-107

[115] Hinrichsen H. et al. (PHV Study Group): Prevalence and risk factors of hepatitis C virus infection in haemodialysis patients: a multicentre study in 2796 patients. Gut, 2002 (51): 429-433

7.3.4.2 HCV Diagnosis in Dialysis Patients[116]

In order to determine an existing HCV infection, testing for anti-HCV and HCV-RNA shall be performed upon referral to dialysis. The above-mentioned study with 2796 patients in 43 German dialysis centres shows that 0.8% of the patients were only HCV-RNA positive. As a result of the disturbed formation of antibodies, uremic patients often become anti-HCV-positive during an HCV infection only after many months and some HCV-RNA positive patients remain anti-HCV-negative for many years. These sources of infection cannot be detected when testing for anti-HCV only is done and the patients are not assigned to the group of those infected with HCV.

To exclude a false positive test result, an HCV confirmation test (mostly Immunoblot or HCV RNA test) shall always be carried out when there is an anti-HCV-positive but HCV-RNA-negative result (about one third of HCV-positive patients). If the anti-HCV can be confirmed positive, then this could hint at a still active as well as an expired infection. For the safety of patients with expired HCV infections who could be re-infected because they lack immunity, a separate dialysis machine shall therefore be used on patients with this constellation of result and a "functional separation" shall take place.

The virus concentration can temporarily fall below the detection limit during chronic HCV infections. In addition, HCV infected dialysis patients show lower HCV concentrations than other HCV infected patients especially immediately after dialysis treatment. An adsorption of the virus in various dialysis membranes has been identified[117, 118]. In addition, Heparin is an inhibitor of the mostly

---

[116] HCV Test: www.kompetenznetz-hepatitis.de/aerzteforum/hep_net/diagnostik.htm

[117] Hayashi H. et al.: Adsorption of hepatitis C virus particles onto the dialyser membrane. Artif. Organs, 1997 (21): 1056-1059

[118] Mizuno M. et al.: Dialysis-membrane-dependent reduction and adsorption of circulating hepatitis C virus during haemodialysis. Nephron, 2002 (91): 235-242

used polymerase chain reaction (PCR) used for confirmation of HCV-RNA which can lead to false negative results. As a consequence, blood samples intended for PCR diagnosis shall, if possible, be taken at a later time after performing heparinisation. Due to these difficulties in detecting HCV-RNA, a subsided expired HCV infection can only be assumed if three HCV-RNA examinations were negative over a period of 12 months.

Usually the sole testing for anti-HCV is sufficient during the semi-annual serological examination for a new HCV infection. An additional examination for HCV-RNA shall be carried out if there is suspicion of a new infection, e.g. if there is evidence that there is a risk of infection outside the dialysis unit, in clarifying an increase of the transaminase, in patients in the same dialysis shift in which a new HCV infection has already been detected. HCV-RNA normally is confirmed positive within 4 weeks after an infection and a few months before the detection of a positive anti-HCV level. As an additional indication for hepatitis infections, the transaminase values GPT and GOT shall be monitored in monthly to quarterly intervals (also see remark ch. 7.3.3.2).

7.3.4.3 HCV Exposure of Staff

An immuno-prophylaxis is not possible after HCV exposure. The transmission of an infection after a needle-stick injury with anti-HCV-positive blood takes place in about 3.0%[119]; here the viral load of the patient has to be taken into consideration. Shall the source of infection in the PCR be negative for HCV-RNA, then the risk of infection is considerably lower.

In case of needle-stick injury, blood shall be squeezed out of the stitch track and disinfection shall follow. Just like after HBV exposure, the injury must be documented. A transmission of the infection has to be ruled out 6 months after the occurrence of

[119] Aktualisierte Empfehlungen 2002 zur beruflichen Exposition mit Blut und biologischen Flüssigkeiten, Fachkomission Klinik und Therapie HIV/AIDS des Bundesamtes für Gesundheit, Bulletin 10: 192-196 und Fragebögen

the injury by means of a negative remaining test for anti-HCV. Alternatively, an infection can be ruled out 3 months after exposure through a negative PCR for HCV-RNA (s. ch. 11.11 HCV Post Exposure Prophylaxis (PEP) for Staff). The measures and the process have to be described in the hygiene plan.

7.3.5 HIV

In 5-10% of the infected patients, a renal involvement develops like an HIV- associated nephropathy of which only a small number of patients becomes subject to dialysis. The HIV-positive patient is extremely immuno-deficient and must be protected from all nosocomial infections.

7.3.5.1 Route of Infection and Risk Factors of HIV Infection

In general, the transmission takes place only through direct contact with blood. Simple contact with the skin does not allow any penetration if the skin is uninjured.

7.3.5.2 HIV Diagnosis in Dialysis Patients

The anti-HIV test is carried out as a screening test for an HIV infection. If the test is positive, it has to be confirmed through a confirmatory test and an additional examination of a second serum sample. Due to the rarity of the infection, control examinations of individual patients are necessary only in cases of persistence or in the event of an individual risk of infection. Annual control examinations of all patients appear to be justified only when HIV infected patients are dialysed in the unit.

7.3.5.3 HIV Exposure of Staff

The risk of infection in case of a percutaneous infection is 0.3% and 0.03% in case of an exposure of the mucosa. The risk of infecting oneself with hepatitis C viruses through needle-stick injuries is about 10 times greater.

7.3.5.4 Post Exposure Prophylaxis after HIV Exposure/PEP

In the event of HIV exposure, a professional and competent office shall always be contacted. Every institution in which HIV-positive patients are dialysed shall have available the telephone number of such a round-the-clock advisory centre in a current alarm plan of the dialysis unit.

Immediately after exposure as well as 6 – 12 – 24 weeks after possible exposure to HIV, HIV AB (antibody) controls have to be carried out.

After exposure to HIV, **documentation** and **registration** has to be done at the professional association.

Action has to be taken immediately after contamination!
(s. ch. 11.8 Post Exposure Prophylaxis (PEP) for Staff)

Needle-stick Injury:
Let bleed out at least 1 minute.
Promote the bleeding through squeezing or spreading the wound if possible.
Leave an antiseptic agent (alcohol-containing skin disinfectant or iodine-containing preparation) on the wound for at least 10 minutes.

Contamination of the Eye:
Wash out the eye with isotonic watery 2.5% PVP iodine solution.
If not available at the moment, wash out with tap water.

Absorption in the Oral Cavity:
Expectorate and rinse with alcohol for disinfection or dilute with tap water if need be.

Drug-based HIV PEP:
Maximum protection will probably only be achieved when drug-based PEP is started within the first 2 hours!
A drug-based PEP is probably ineffective if it takes place later than 72 hours after an exposure of the mucosa or later than 24 hours after a percutaneous or iv. exposure respectively.
In case of doubts, one can also start with urgently administering the first PEP medication immediately.
The choice of measures depends among others on the pre-treatment of the source of infection, e.g. possible resistance of the HIV against drugs already used in the therapy, possible cross-resistances of the virus, new drugs coming on the market.
The drug-based PEP shall be carried out for 28 days while controlling the laboratory values like the haemogram, transaminase, AP, gamma-glutamyl transferase, creatinine, and urea.
A termination of the prophylaxis is possible at any time if it appears to be unnecessary because of the circumstances and the course of events leading to the accident.
Indications on how to start drug-based PEP are given in ch. 11.9.[120, 121]

7.3.6 Multi-Resistant Pathogens in Dialysis

7.3.6.1 Definition

Only 10 years after the discovery of penicillin, 80% of the bacteria were resistant against the preparation. The increase of multimorbid risk patients with an increased predisposition for

[120] Empfehlungen zur HIV-Postexpositionsprophylaxe (www.rki.de)
[121] Postexpositionelle Prophylaxe der HIV-Exposition/PEP, Deutsch-Österreichische Empfehlungen (www.rki.de)

infections especially in intensive care units, the non-specific and frequently combined use of antibiotics, the use of antibiotics in animal feed and the world-wide exchange of germs through travelling activities and global transport of consumer goods facilitated the formation of multi-resistant pathogens in the last decades.

A Methicillin-resistant Staphylococcus aureus (MRSA) is known since the end of the 80s. Alarmingly, first cases of resistance have also been coming up recently against so-called reserve antibiotics:

VISA = Vancomycin intermediate Staphylococcus aureus
VRSA = Vancomycin-resistant Staphylococcus aureus
VRE = Vancomycin-resistant Enterococcus
MRE = Methicillin (multi-)resistant Enterococcus

In the daily routine of dialysis, mainly the outbreak of MRSA has till now been of importance. Therefore the following information refers to the procedure related to MRSA.

7.3.6.2 Meaning[122, 123]

40% of the population show a "normal" settlement of Staphylococcus aureus, and even up to 65% among hospital employees. For persons with healthy immune defence, MRSA strains are generally not infectious or more dangerous than antibiotic-sensitive strains[124].

---

[122] RKI-Empfehlung: Empfehlung zur Prävention und Kontrolle von Methicillin-resistenten Staphylococcus aureus (MRSA)-Stämmen in Krankenhäusern und anderen medizinischen Einrichtungen. Bundesgesundheitsbl – Gesundheitsforsch – Gesundheitsschutz, 1999 (42): 954-958 (www.rki.de)

[123] RKI: Kommentar zu den „Empfehlungen zur Prävention und Kontrolle von Methicillin-resistenten Staphylococcus aureus-Stämmen in Krankenhäusern und anderen medizinischen Einrichtungen. Epidemiologisches Bulletin Nr. 2004) (46): 396 (www.rki.de)

[124] RKI: Zur MRSA-Situation in Deutschland im Jahr 2003. Epidemiologisches Bulletin 2004 (42): 358-361 (www.rki.de)

For dialysis patients whose defence systems are weak, life-threatening clinical characteristics like bacteraemia or sepsis can develop from skin infections like erysipelas, furunculosis, panaritium or infections of the shunts for example.

7.3.6.3 Route of Infection

In the body, Staphylococcus aureus is mainly found in the vestibules of the nose and other wet parts of the body, e.g. axillae, groin, pillory borders, perineum. The transmission to open wounds usually takes place by means of direct contact during manual manipulations and is seldom organic.

7.3.6.4 Diagnosis/Screening

Those to be considered as risk groups within in-hospital dialysis are first and foremost elderly patients, e.g. from nursing homes, diabetics, patients with gangrene or varicose ulcer, patients during or after longer periods of hospitalisation as well as after long-term antibiotic therapy.

Regular inspection of the feet is not only of special importance to diabetics. Due to the fact that during foot visitations or care activities for diabetic feet the spreading of resistant pathogens cannot be excluded, these activities shall be performed outside of treatment room before or after the dialysis treatment. Ambulatory services have to be informed about the risk factors for transmission.

Regular bacteriological screening by means of swab examinations shall be considered for risk groups, possibly also as preliminary screening during the initial contact e.g. within the context of transferring and/or if there was a lack of prior information. Due to the fact that hospitals and institutions performing ambulatory operations are obliged to record and evaluate nosocomial infections and the outbreak of pathogens with special resistance and multiresistance in accordance with § 23 of the Infections Protection Act

(IfSG), this often problematic deficit of information will probably be corrected soon.

First of all, bacteriological examinations of the suspicious localisation, e.g. wounds are necessary. If the MRSA diagnosis is positive, the areas of the body prone to contamination have to be bacteriologically examined for colonisation/infection, e.g.:

- both vestibules of the nose
- pharynx
- forehead-pilary border
- both armpits
- perineum/groins
- urine (above all during urine drainage)

7.3.6.5 Prevention of the Transmission of Infections[125]

The most important measure of prophylaxis against infection is the **DISINFECTION OF HANDS** which as the basis of hygiene and therefore education of staff and patients has to take place regularly and has to be monitored.

MRSA/MRE colonised or infected patients have to be treated separately from other patients in a separate treatment room. In order to keep the organisational efforts reasonable, the MRSA patients shall be assigned to a room which is exclusively used for the treatment of this group of patients. The room shall be located within the shortest distance and possibly, no other treatment section shall be crossed on the way. Consumables shall be stored close to and prepared in the room only for the individual patient and for immediate use.

Remark:
The assignment of a separate dialysis machine is not necessary. A dialysis machine which was used on MRSA/MRE patients must not undergo the special disinfec-

[125] Dettenkofer M. et al.: Bewertung unterschiedlicher Hygienekonzepte zur Kontrolle von MRSA. DIMDI 2003 (http://gripsdb.dimdi.de)

tion measures like is done with machines used on patients infected with HBV and HCV.

Remark:
If the institution is provided with an isolation unit, it can be used for MRSA patients. An isolation unit[126] is a separate treatment section which can be reached directly by patients, i.e. without passing through the non-infectious section. The isolation section is provided with all the necessary adjoining rooms, e.g. lock, monitoring section, wet workroom, tea kitchen if necessary, patients' WC, if necessary staff WC, wardrobe, store for sterile goods. As this section represents an independent unit, a corresponding number of nurses have to be assigned to it. The former "yellow sections" are suitable as an isolation unit if no other patients are taken care of there at the time of the "MRSE/MRE dialysis".

Other patients can also be treated here before and after if in between a scrub and wet disinfection of horizontal surfaces which are near to the patients, the machines as well as the working surfaces and floors is performed using confirmed agents and procedures.

Operational Measures

As staff normally moves between the MRSA room and the other sections of treatment, high requirements for the observance of the hygiene measures have to be made:

- When entering the treatment room, staff has to put on protective aprons, mouth/nose protection as well as disposable examination gloves.
- Bed with mattress (recommended to be fluid-proof, protective cover with disinfectable surface), floor, horizontal surfaces and dialysis machines have to undergo a scrub/wet disinfection between the treatments.
- Devices like stethoscopes, blood pressure cuffs, tourniquet and all other nursing tools shall be assigned exclusively to the MRSA/MRE patients and shall likewise be disinfected after every treatment.

[126] Cooper B.S. et al.: Isolation measures in the hospital management of Methicillin-resistant Staphylococcus aureus (MRSA): systematic review of the literature. BMJ Vol. 2004 (329): 533-542 (www.bmj.com)

- Reusable crockery can be used if the used crockery can be brought to the disinfecting dishwasher (validated procedure) in a transport container which can be disinfected both inside and outside. If this is not possible, then disposable crockery shall be used.
- Sterile goods and dressing material are to be prepared patient-related.
- The gloves as well as the mouth/nose protection shall be put in the waste bag before leaving the treatment room.
- The protective overall has to be taken off and kept in the treatment anteroom before leaving the treatment unit.
- A hygienic disinfection of the hands has to be done after this.
- The protective overall has to be put in a tightly sealable laundry bag – also using the double bag method – at the end of the shift at the latest. In case of disposable overalls, a tightly sealable laundry bag shall be used also applying the double bag method.
- After every dialysis, blankets, pillows and their covers have to be disinfected and reprocessed just like in normal hospital laundry. The dirty linen has to be collected in a tightly sealable laundry bag and sent sealed to the laundry also using the double bag method. Devices may only leave the isolation unit after preliminary disinfection.
- Waste is collected in the treatment unit and as long as no other factors have to be respected, it is sealed also using the double bag method and then put into the domestic rubbish (s. ch. 11.2).
- The treatment unit has to be clearly marked as such (e.g. "Visitors please contact the nursing service").

Patient-Related Measures in Case of a Colonisation of the Pharynx and/or Body Parts

- Upon entering the dialysis unit the patient carries out a hygienic disinfection of the hands under supervision.
- Upon entering the dialysis unit the patient puts on mouth/nose protection and a protective overall.

- The patient is brought to his treatment room using the shortest route and if possible without crossing other treatment sections. The patient can take off the protective overall as well as the mouth and nose protection in the treatment room.
- So long as the patient uses a WC, a scrub-wet disinfection has to be done afterwards. To be disinfected are:
  - toilet bowl with seat
  - floor
  - walls within the splashing section (ca. 1.5 m radius)
  - hand basin including the fittings
- In case MRSA is detected in the urine, he shall be assigned his own toilet as soon as possible.
- Before leaving the treatment room, the patient carries out a hygienic disinfection of the hands.
- Before leaving the room, the patient puts on a fresh mouth/nose protection as well as a fresh apron.

Patient-Related Measures in Case of Wound Colonisation without the Participation of the Naso-pharynx or Other Body Parts

Patients with non-oozing and properly attended dressings do not need to be room-separated. They shall however be functionally isolated respecting the operational measures:

- Before the dialysis treatment, a change of dressing shall be carried out in a separate room if necessary and a scrub-wet disinfection done afterwards.
- The dressing shall be covered.
- The dressing shall not be opened during the dialysis.
- When changing the dressing, the medical staff shall wear mouth/nose protection, disposable gloves, and protective overalls. After changing the dressing, the disposable gloves and mouth/nose protection have to be put in a properly sealable rubbish bag, while the protective overall shall be put in a properly sealable laundry bag using the double bag method too; a disinfection of the hands is necessary afterwards.

- The patient must carry out a hygienic disinfection of the hands before entering and when leaving the treatment section.
- In order to successfully to eradicate bacteria from a patient, it is necessary after every dialysis to process the blankets, pillows and their covers like normal hospital laundry using disinfectants. The use of washable disinfectable blankets is recommended.
- Regular swabs of the surrounding wound area and the naso-pharynx are carried out. If the diagnosis is positive, a spatially separated treatment is necessary.

7.3.6.6 Transport of Patients

In accordance with the guideline of the RKI[127], there is no risk of infection by an MRSA-colonised patient to healthy persons through the usual social contacts especially outside the medical facility. He can therefore use public transportation as well as a taxi.

Due to the increased infection risks of dialysis patients, the joint transport of an MRSA-colonised patient and a non-colonised dialysis patient has to be rejected.

For transport in ambulances, the responsible staff has to be informed about the colonisation/infection of a dialysis patient in order to be able to initiate the appropriate measures defined in the rescue service[128] department. Wound infections and lesions of MRSA patients have to be tightly covered. MRSA patients with naso-pharyngeal colonisation must wear mouth/nose protection during transport.

---

[127] RKI-Empfehlung: Empfehlung zur Prävention und Kontrolle von Methicillin-resistenten Staphylococcus aureus (MRSA)-Stämmen in Krankenhäusern und anderen medizinischen Einrichtungen. Bundesgesundheitsbl – Gesundheits-forsch – Gesundheitsschutz, 1999 (42): 954-958 (www.rki.de)

[128] RKI: Anforderungen der Hygiene an den Krankentransport in Krankenkraft-wagen. Bundesgesundheitsblatt, 1989 (32): 169-170 (www.rki.de)

7.3.6.7 Remediation of the MRSA Carrier

Remediation has to be striven for, however there are at present various possible strategies and ways which are being discussed controversially[129].
With the help of a defined protocol of procedure, all the important steps can be carried out and monitored (s. ch. 11.14 MRSA Infection – protocol of procedures).

7.3.6.8 Control Examinations after Remediation Measures

Patients

The remediation is successful when three consecutive swabs from three consecutive dialysis sessions are MRSA/MRE-negative.
Transferred to the special situation of ambulatory dialysis, e.g. if the patient is in the institution every 2-3 days, the following procedure is recommended:

A Swabs testing shall be done at the end of the remediation on three consecutive dialysis days (first swab after > 24 hrs and < 48 hrs)

B Next control phase after the confirmation of the negative results (A all negative) after 30 days

C Further control swabs during dialysis treatment after 3 months and in case of suspected re-infection.

D In case of a positive MRSA diagnosis, the remediation is continued immediately during a period of up to 10 days if necessary and isolation shall be maintained.

Successfully decontaminated patients can then be treated again in the non-infectious section.
During the remediation of wound colonisation or local skin colonisation, control swabs shall also be done in the vestibule of the nose in order to examine the success of the treatment.

---

[129] Werner, H.-P.; Hygiene Institut der Johannes-Gutenberg-Universität Mainz: Die mikrobiozide Wirksamkeit ausgewählter Antiseptika. Hygiene und Medizin, mhp-Verlag 02/1992

Remark:
The half-life period has to be observed if during or parallel to the remediation, Vancomycin administered intravenously or orally is used for pursuing other therapeutic goals. The interval for the control swabs has to be undertaken in agreement with the treating physician.

7.3.6.9 Diagnostic Screening in Cases of Frequent Outbreaks of MRSA in Institutions

Frequent outbreaks of MRSA means: There is a detection in many patients (> 2) which is correlated in terms of space and timely occurrence and exhibits a clonal identity. In this case, screening by means of swabbing the vestibules of the nose and pharynx of all the patients in the treatment unit concerned as well as of the medical staff who had direct contact with the MRSA patients shall be done. The examination of the staff shall be done by the company physician. If there is colonisation, a remediation therapy shall be recommended. Employees with a nasal colonisation of MRSA/MRE like physicians and nurses for example, are only allowed to continue working in direct patient care after a remediation therapy.

The therapy is successful if after remediation measures 3 swabs done on three consecutive days or on 3 dialysis days on patients (first swab after > 24 hrs and < 48 hrs) are MRSA-negative thereby confirming the success of the treatment. Further controls have to be carried out after 1 month and 3 months.

7.3.6.10 Circulation of Information, Enlightenment and Duty of Notification

All the persons concerned with care and treatment, e.g. ward physicians, clinic staff, general practitioners, dentists, dialysis physicians and dialysis nurses, etc. must be immediately informed about the diagnosis and they shall regularly exchange information about the state of the treatment.

The patient, relatives and other persons in his environment shall be included in all the steps from the very beginning (s. ch. 11.13 Information Sheet for MRSA Patients).

There is no duty of notification of MRSA patients in case of sporadic outbreaks according to the Infections Protection Act. However, if there are frequent outbreaks of nosocomial infections in which an epidemic connection is probable or suspected, this has to be reported immediately to the public health department without reporting it as an outbreak[130].

7.3.7 Infectious Gastroenteritis

The pathogens of infectious gastroenteritis are various viruses and bacteria, e.g. noro-viruses, rota viruses, salmonella species or Staphylococcus aureus[131].

According to § 6 of the Infections Prevention Act (IfSG), there is a duty of notification in case of suspicion of and illness from microbial-induced food poisoning or an acute infectious gastroenteritis if:

- a person is concerned who is entrusted with the manufacture, treatment or distribution of food
- a person is concerned who works in the kitchen of restaurants and other institutions where canteen meals are served
- two or more similar illnesses in which an epidemic connection is probable or suspected appear at the same time

According to § 42 of the Infections Protection Act (IfSG) (occupational prohibition and ban on employment), all persons who are sick or suspected of being infected with an infectious gastroenteritis are not supposed to work or be employed in areas where food is handled.
The transmission route is faecal-oral or through air-borne infection when vomiting. Depending on the particular pathogen, the incu-

130 IfSG § 6 Abs. 3
131 RKI-Ratgeber Infektionskrankheiten – Merkblätter für Ärzte (www.rki.de)

bation period is 1-3 days. The required hygienic measures and the special requirements for the selection of disinfectants can be taken from ch. 11.12 "Hygiene Measures during Infectious Illnesses".

7.3.8 Tuberculosis

7.3.8.1 Meaning

Tuberculosis is in the first place an aerogenous transmissible infectious disease and still a global health problem with a traditionally known socio-economical background. Worldwide, lung tuberculosis is the most widespread infectious disease caused by bacteria and resulting in death even though nowadays efficient diagnosis and successful therapy (at least for uncomplicated tuberculosis) is quite possible. At present there are no consistent European standards for the evaluation of disinfection procedures in dialysis machines. The effectiveness has to be verified or evidenced by the manufacturers within the framework of the admissions procedure of medical devices. The operator can request the corresponding expert's report from the manufacturer.

Lung tuberculosis is caused by the Mycobacterium tuberculosis as well as the typical mycobacteria like M. africanum and M. bovis belonging to the Mycobacterium tuberculosis complex. The incubation period may be several weeks. Infectious patients are those who are apparently sick or latently infected who by means of bacteria-loaded (i.e. especially minute alveolar-permeable and slowly sedimenting) droplets expel tubercle bacilli in high concentration with the sputum/respiratory secretion. Mycobacteria are diagnosed in a specialised laboratory as acid-resistant rods in so-called microscopic (coloured) direct preparations (lower detection limit: 5000-10000 bacteria/ml). The detection by sample culturing with a detection limit of 10-100 bacteria/ml including the resistance patterns usually takes several weeks.

Open tuberculosis is present if the tubercular bacteria can be dispersed outside the body when a tubular cavity becomes connected to the bronchial system for example. The term "open" lung tuberculosis is independent of the concentration of bacteria and intensity of infection.
The number of new infections and the mortality rate in many developing countries and especially in the former Eastern Bloc countries is increasingly rising including the incidences and the dissemination of multi-resistant M. tuberculosis strains, so-called MDR-TB germs (i.e. at least resistant against isoniazid and rifampicin, MDR = multi drug resistant). This leads to limited success of treatment and also to increased health risk for the nursing staff.

7.3.8.2 Prevention

The aim must be to identify a dialysis patient with tuberculosis as early as possible to initiate all necessary hygienically relevant measures for isolation and prevention of other patients and staff and to implement (execute) specific tuberculostatic treatment on behalf of the individual patient and public health.

Remark:
According to the hygiene plan required in § 36 of the Infections Protection Act (IfSG), a dialysis unit can set its own measures for cases of TB.

In all the situations stated below, already in case of suspicion, a microbiological clarification, the rapid consultation of a tuberculosis specialist or the involvement of a hospital hygienist and/or the responsible qualified hygienist is absolutely necessary.
The close co-operation with the admitting or attending physician and (if necessary) the family and other persons concerned is also advisable.
The regulations of Infections Protection Act (IfSG) §§ 6, 8 and 9, request obligatory notification of the responsible public health department within 24 hours in case of confirmed tuberculosis requiring therapy.

7.3.8.3 Recognising the Risk Groups

The risk of occurrence of tuberculosis in a dialysis treatment section is either due to reactivation of latent tuberculosis under specific circumstances such as immunosuppression during transplantation, HIV infection/AIDS or other severe illness or by admission of new patients with a risk anamnesis. Relevant data to be collected for the risk anamnesis are the country of origin, the social status, the prevalence of tuberculosis in the case history of the patient and/or in the family. All these factors are important for risk anamnesis.

7.3.8.4 Consequences and Measures

Patients with Tuberculosis of Lung or Larynx requiring treatment

The detection of acid-resistant rods in the direct microscopic sputum/sputum sample of the patient has not yet been confirmed. There is a risk of transmission when the required hygienic measures for protection are not implemented.

General Guidelines for prevention of infection:

- Spatial separation and all material to be used patient-specific
- Door of treatment room shall always be closed, there shall be a sign on the door, e.g. "Consultants and visitors please first report to the ward office before entering the room"
- All internal and external staff must be informed
- Wearing of appropriate mouth/nose protection with valve by the patient and staff during activities that are near to the face/head which can cause aerosols and the wearing of protective glasses by the staff
- Protective gloves and protective overalls in case of possible contact with excretions, secretions, body fluids, infectious body parts or contaminated objects
- Executing of a hygienic disinfection of the hands after taking off the gloves
- Changing the protective apron per shift

- Wearing of qualitative high-grade mouth/nose protection without valve by the patient within the dialysis unit, outside of his treatment room and for the transportation with an ambulance
- Diagnostic, therapeutic or nursing measures inducing coughing or other types of aerosol formation, e.g. bronchoscopy, gastroscopy, dentist, only in case of clinical emergency and under special protection of the staff with special high-quality particle mask with valve (FFP2 mask) as mouth and nose protection, protective glasses

Disinfection, Cleaning, Waste Disposal:

A hygienic disinfection of the hands is necessary before and after entering the room, before and after contact with the patient, after getting into contact with germ-containing materials, and after removing gloves. Regarding the effectiveness against TB, the manufacturers' information has to be respected.
The disinfection of the surfaces including the floor takes place after the end of the treatment with surface disinfectants approved by experts as being effective against TB.
The cleaning staff has to be instructed accurately. They have to wear mouth/nose protection, protective overalls, and protective gloves. The room shall be cleaned last. Cleaning trolleys shall remain out of the room.
Visible contamination with blood, secretions, excretions etc. shall be immediately removed using disinfectants.
Instruments are to be carried to the disinfection automate in a closed box which can be disinfected both from outside and inside or have to be disinfected in the treatment room by means of a plunge bath.
Textiles are to be placed in a laundry bag in the room. For transportation they are to be put in an additional laundry bag. The reprocessing is performed as stated for infectious hospital laundry.
Potential pathogen-containing materials have to be disposed of separately as group C waste (AS 180103 infectious waste).

Used crockery has to be treated the same way a crockery from MRSA patients (s. ch. 7.3.6).

Patients with lung and/or laryngeal tuberculosis confirmed in a direct microscopic sputum

Due to the risk of transmission and a possible MDR TB, the dialysis treatment shall be performed in a special clinic.

Patients with extrapulmonary tuberculosis of the organs (urogenital TB, lymphatic nodes TB, bone-TB, skin-TB, tuberculosis meningitis).

There is only a minimal risk of transmission if all the general rules of hygiene are respected.
The medical staff have to be informed.
Spatial separation is only necessary when secretion of infectious material, e.g. wound secretions, urine, peritoneal fluids etc. is to be expected.
When disposing urine from patients with urogenital tuberculosis, it is absolutely necessary to wear protective gloves and a fluid-proof protective apron as well as mouth/nose protection. The disposal takes place in a bed-pan cleaning system, providing thermal disinfection.
In a dialysis patient peritoneal tuberculosis treated with PD therapy, the used solution will be disposed of in the sink of the waste disposal room. Above-mentioned protective measures apply correspondingly.
During unavoidable care of drained lesions, e.g. with lymph node tuberculosis, the staff have to wear mouth/nose protection, disposable protective gloves and fluid-proof protective aprons. As a rule, no manipulations shall be done on the freshly applied dressing of a TB wound during the dialysis session.

Patients with a previously unidentified open and untreated lung tuberculosis that have already been dialysed in the institution

The responsible public health department, the company physician and if necessary the hospital hygienist have to be consulted immediately. Their instructions or recommendations have to be followed.

A final disinfection is performed on the orders of the public health department and/or after consultation with the hygienist.

7.3.9 Parasitosis

Parasitosis like scabies for example is acquiring an increasing importance in ambulatory dialysis. Extensive information can be obtained from the homepage of the Robert Koch Institute in Berlin in case of need.[132]

7.3.10 Forms of Isolation

Isolation measures aim at interrupting the dissemination routes of pathogens through specific behaviour and spatial measures. On the other hand, they can also be necessary if an immuno-deficient patient himself has to be protected from infections.

The isolation measures to be applied depend on:
- the infectivity of the pathogen
- the route of transmission
- the danger to the patients
- the danger which emanates from the patients

[132] www.rki.de

Standard Isolation

Standard isolation is carried out for diseases that can be transmitted only through direct contact or contact with infective secretions and excretions.

Cohort Isolation

The setting is the same as in standard isolation, but in this case, many patients with equal spectrum of pathogens are treated in the same room.

Functional Isolation

It describes an isolation which concentrates on the specific hygienic behaviour during all nursing/medical interventions by the employees as well as the use of patient-specific equipment/ dialysis machines. Functional isolation does not require any spatial isolation. In this case, the main issue is to prevent infection from the hands of staff performing the treatment as well as pathogen transmission through material by patient specific use of materials.

Treatment of patients with hepatitis C can be referred to as an example for the treatment in the dialysis section.

Protective Isolation (Reverse Isolation)

Protective isolation protects the patient from pathogens in his surroundings. Everything that the patient has contact with shall be sterile or close to sterile. Everything that comes from the patient is disposed of with the household waste. The procedure is the same like in strict isolation, only in the reverse sense. Items and equipment for nursing care shall be used patient-specific.

8 Catering

8.1 Goal and Rationale

Foodstuffs are to be stored, prepared and distributed in such a way that their consumption is safe for a person's health and appetising as well. Harmful influences on food can e.g. be caused by micro-organisms, insects, steams, smoke, aerosols, light, heat and cold, air and other gases, waste, liquid waste, chemicals, smells, climatic influences as well as human and animal secretions.

8.2 Hygienic Requirements for the Supply of Food to Patients

Foodstuffs provide perfect conditions for the growth of many pathogens, therefore many special requirements have to be made during the supply of food

- on staff
- on structural and organisational conditions
- on handling of food.

The requirements based on the Foodstuffs Hygiene Ordinance (LMHV) and the Infection Protection Act (IfSG) are given in detail in the following:

These requirements apply irrespective of the chosen supply system, e.g.:

- for the preparation of self-made sandwiches
- for distribution of prepared sandwiches which have been delivered, if these are not separately packed but stored in the kitchen, repacked or served on plates
- for distributing deep-frozen meals, that have been heated in the in-house kitchen
- for portioning and distributing meals delivered warm (in so-called "thermoports" or electric food warmers)

Additional requirements in accordance with § 4 of the Foodstuffs Hygiene Ordinance (LMHV) can be necessary if meals are self-produced in the kitchen of the dialysis unit, this could be the introduction of a self-monitoring system based on the principles of the HACCP concept (Hazard Analysis and Critical Control Points). If the dialysis unit is located within a clinic and the patients' food is supplied by the hospital kitchen, e.g. with covered tableware when packed lunch is handed out to the patients, then most of the requirements are unnecessary.

8.3 Requirements on Staff

For persons who are not in possession of a health certificate in accordance with § 18 of the Federal Epidemic Control Act (BSeuchG), according to § 43 sect. 1 of the Infections Protection Act (IfSG) and who are entrusted with producing, handling and bringing foodstuffs into circulation, participation in a singular introduction course is mandatory before commencing work. These instructions are to be given by a representative of the public health department or a physician engaged by the public health department and will instruct about regulations regarding forbiddance of temporary or permanent execution of this job.

Independent of this, according to §§ 42, 43 of the Infections Protection Act (IfSG) the operator of the dialysis unit has to instruct and teach this group of staff annually on how to deal with foodstuffs in accordance with the Foodstuffs Hygiene Ordinance (LMHV) as well as the regulations on temporary or permanent ban to execute this job.

Participation in these instructions and education is a precondition for the employment of these persons in areas where foodstuffs are handled. This participation has to be documented in written form. The responsibility for instructing and education of staff of external companies that are in charge of delivering the food is with their employers.

The education or instruction about temporary or permanent ban to execute this job implies that persons who produce, handle or bring foodstuffs into circulation are not allowed to execute their job, if they show symptoms indicating one of the following conditions or if such symptoms have been diagnosed by a physician:

- Diarrhoea with sudden onset, e.g. acute infectious gastroenteritis, viral hepatitis A or E.
- Skin diseases or infected skin lesions with pathogens, that could be transmitted via food.

Symptoms indicating the above-mentioned diseases, e.g.:

- Diarrhoea with loose stool, as well as nausea, vomiting and fever
- Fever with serious headache, abdominal pain or joint pain and constipation (serious diarrhoea starts only after some days).
- Jaundice of the skin and eyeballs with weakness and loss of appetite.

Occurrence of these symptoms has to be reported immediately to the employer.

Till clarification of symptoms and diagnosis the person concerned is prohibited to execute his/her job in catering services for patients.

If the person affected does not feel ill still prohibition to handle foodstuffs persists if one of the following pathogens is found in a sample of his/her faecal matter:

- Salmonellae
- Shigella
- Enteropathic Escherichia coli (EHEC)
- Cholera vibrio

8.4 Requirements on Staff Hygiene

Persons who produce, handle or bring foodstuffs into circulation must pay particular attention to appropriate hygiene of body and clothing.

- Before starting work jewellery on hands and forearms has to be removed.
- Fingernails of employees are to be clean, trimmed short and not painted.
- Before commencing work, after visiting the toilet, cleaning nose and other unclean activities, hands are to be disinfected.
- When dealing with open foodstuffs, hair has to be covered with a headgear.
- Smoking, eating and drinking in the kitchen is forbidden.
- Kitchen staff has to change work clothes daily. To avoid transmission of any pathogens from the treatment section into the kitchen, work clothes of the kitchen staff have to be covered with a protective gown before entering treatment rooms. This protective gown is to be kept outside of the kitchen or in the front section of it.
- If nurses are involved in the preparation and/or distribution of food, the protective gown which is worn during patient treatment has to be taken off before entering the kitchen. The medical staff is not allowed to enter the kitchen in their work clothes if those are not covered with a protective gown during the direct care and treatment of patients and work and handling in treatment sections.
- Skin lesions on hands shall be covered with a waterproof plaster, using a dressing with finger stall or gloves have to be worn.
- Diseases like diarrhoea and/or vomiting have to be reported immediately to the management of the institution and shall be medically clarified and diagnosed.

8.5 Hygienic Requirements regarding Structural and Organisational Conditions

Kitchens used for the supply of patients shall be constructed in such a way that the regulations for foodstuffs hygiene can be adhered to and protection of foodstuffs against detrimental influences can be assured.

Citation of the Foodstuffs Hygiene Ordinance (LMHV): "Surfaces including surfaces of equipment which come into contact with foodstuffs have to be maintained in an impeccable state and have to be easy to clean and disinfect, when necessary".

Cleaning and disinfection procedures of the kitchen have to be executed according to the disinfection plan set up for the kitchen section.

For Germany, solely disinfectants recommended by the German Society for Veterinary Medicine (DVG)[133] are to be used. This is to guarantee that the disinfectants used, do not have a negative effect on the foodstuffs, but still fulfil the special requirements for disinfection purposes in kitchen areas, namely increased fat and protein load and disinfection at low temperatures. The instructions for use of the disinfectant manufacturers have to be followed.

- Waste water resulting from disinfection and cleaning procedures has to be disposed of outside of the kitchen if a separate sink is not available.
- All working utensils, e.g. knives, cutting boards, slicing machines are to be out of components that can withstand disinfection. No working materials with wooden components are to be used.
- The tableware of the patients has to be placed directly in the disinfecting dishwasher and has to be processed without it first

[133] Deutsche Veterinärmedizinische Gesellschaft (DVG): www.dvg.net

being put on clean working surfaces. Regular testing for microbiological effectiveness is to be carried out with biological indicators to ensure the disinfecting effect of the dishwasher.

- All refrigerating and freezing appliances are equipped with thermometers.
- A hand basin with dispensers for disinfectant and soap as well as paper towels is available separately from the sink. If this is not the case, the sink serves as a hand basin. No cleaning work is to be done here.
- Unclean working procedures (working with dirty crockery, waste disposal and cleaning works) are to be spatially separated from clean working procedures (preparation of meals). If this is not possible, the working surfaces have to be cleaned and disinfected after unclean activities and before performing clean activities (chronological and organisational separation).
- Windows in the kitchen section that can be opened, are equipped with wire mesh, that can be removed easily for cleaning purposes.
- Windows within the immediate vicinity of clean working surfaces shall not have any curtains or interior blinds.
- There shall be no plants in the kitchen.
- The kitchen door has to be kept closed. Unauthorised persons (patients, cab drivers, medical staff wearing clothes which are worn during treatment of patients) have no access to the kitchen.
- The kitchen is not to be used for other purposes, for example as staff lounge. If that is not possible, organisational measures (like defining break times for staff) have to ensure that the kitchen is not used as staff lounge when meals are being prepared
- Waste bins are to be kept closed and shall be opened without hand contact.
- Waste bins have to be emptied daily.

8.6 Hygienic Requirements for Handling Foodstuffs

These include all measures to be taken in order to prevent a detrimental influence on food

- during purchase and delivery
- during storage
- during preparation
- during serving of meals

A reception control of all goods and foodstuff after purchase by in-house staff or after delivery through a service provider (caterer, large kitchen, wholesale market, and butcher among others) has to take place and is to be documented.

The reception control can include:

- Best-before date and optical status of the goods
- Hygienic status of packaging, freight container respectively
- Monitoring of the minimum temperatures[134] of the goods
- < –18 °C for frozen foods
- +65 °C for warm meals
- < +7 °C for sausage and cheese
- The temperature is to be monitored with an appropriate food thermometer (insertion thermometer). The insertion thermometer has to be cleaned and disinfected with an alcoholic disinfectant after each use.
- Temperature monitoring is not necessary if foodstuff is supplied in a delivery van for refrigerated or frozen goods, if the van is equipped with a thermograph and printouts of the readings are randomly checked.

In case of self-**purchase** of perishable foodstuffs e.g. by kitchen staff or auxiliary staff, observance of the cold chain has to be ensured. Therefore foodstuffs have to be transported to the dialysis centre as quickly as possible. Cool boxes or insulated containers

[134] Bundesinstitut für gesundheitlichen Verbraucherschutz und Veterinärmedizin (BgVV): Merkblatt: Temperaturanforderungen und -empfehlungen für Lebensmittel. 1999 (www.bgvv.de)

have to be used for transportation of cooled or frozen foodstuffs. Thermometers are to be placed in these containers. The temperature in the freight containers has to be documented when delivering the foodstuffs.

Stored foodstuff has to be checked regularly to avoid detrimental effects on food.

This has to be documented. Criteria to be checked include e.g.:
- Monitoring on work days of the storage temperature in refrigerators and freezers.
- Food packages that were repacked or opened but not completely used up have to be labelled with the best-by date of the original package. Leftovers are to be stored in the refrigerator or freezer respectively.
- Prepared food e.g. sandwiches are solely distributed on the same day.
- Cleaning agents and disinfectants are stored separately from foodstuffs.

During **preparation and distribution of meals,** the following has to be observed:
- Before preparation and distribution of foodstuffs, best-before dates have to be checked and respected.
- Sandwiches have to be distributed immediately after preparation or delivery. If this is not possible, they have to be covered and stored while monitoring the intended storage temperature.
- Frozen foods shall not be unfrozen before heating. Thawed food has to be disposed off. During the distribution of heated meals, **checks of the core temperature** (> 65 °C) have to be carried out randomly and must be documented.
- Warm delivered food (large kitchen, caterer) has to be kept warm at a temperature of > 65 °C using appropriate measures like heating trolleys until serving. This has to be checked **(at the time of serving)** and documented.
- In case of self-preparation of food, additional requirements in accordance with § 4 of the Foodstuffs Hygiene Ordinance (LMHV) can become necessary; e.g. the introduction of a

self-monitoring system based on the principles of the HACCP concept.

The parameters to be examined as well as the intervals of examination must be clearly defined in the hygiene plan.

To guarantee performance of good practice in foodstuffs hygiene on the long term, staff members involved in preparation and distribution of food have to be educated on the subject of foodstuffs hygiene in accordance with § 4 sect. 2 of the Foodstuffs Hygiene Ordinance (LMHV) on a regular basis. The content of the education can be orientated towards the DIN 10514 "Foodstuffs Hygiene and Hygiene Education".

9 Waste Management

9.1 Goal and Rationale

Staff safety has highest priority at disposal and management of waste. The risk of infection when handling waste arises mainly from activities which imply close contact with patients and/or patients materials. Waste transportation pathways in dialysis units have to be as short as possible and the waste containers must provide sufficient protection from contamination and infection.

9.2 Legal Basis and Recommendations for Waste Management

There are numerous regulations for the disposal of solid waste. Among the many complexes of regulations (laws, ordinances, guidelines, and instruction leaflets), the most important are:

- the Recycling Management and Waste Law (KrW-/AbfG)
- the Waste Catalogue Ordinance (AVV)
- the Ordinance about the verification of waste disposal (NachwV)
- the "Directive on the proper disposal of waste from facilities of the public health service" of the state working group "waste" (LAGA) of January 2002

Local regulations for disposal may always be important and need to be considered.

9.3 Type and Origin of Wastes

Up to 4 kg of waste with a volume of up to 40 l is produced during each dialysis treatment session in Germany. The total annual volume of waste resulting from dialysis treatment comes to ca. 280,000 m^3.

These include used dialysers and blood lines, additional materials used in dialysis like syringes, cannulae, disposable gloves and pads.

The other remaining wastes from dialysis treatments are packaging materials. This fraction is full of recycling potential.

The LAGA instructions for classification of waste from dialysis are recommended. Statements made concerning the classification of medical wastes in the categories "non-infectious" or "infectious" were considered and interpreted by the working group. Legally correct categorisation and disposal of waste, is beyond the scope of this guideline and the following statement is only with regard to the categorisation and disposal of medical waste resulting directly from dialysis treatment.

The classification of waste to a waste code in this guideline is carried out according to the criteria of the Waste Catalogue Ordinance (AVV). Waste codes with "asterix" have to be disposed of as hazardous waste. Mandatory waste consignment as well as the observance of the legal regulations on hazardous goods is required.

Remark:
It is assumed that in regular dialysis operations the amount of residual blood is limited to approx. 1 ml within the blood lines and dialyser after rinse back with saline. The risk of an infectious transmission through dialysers and blood lines from the treatment of infectious patients can not be compared to the risk arising from blood-filled vessel or blood-soaked waste which is mentioned in the LAGA instruction leaflet.

The disposal of a dialyser and/or blood line which is filled with undiluted blood, is an exceptional situation. As mentioned above regularly rinsed back used dialysers and blood lines from treatment of HBV/HCV or HIV-positive patients can be disposed of together with the waste from code 18 01 04.

9.4 Classification of Waste Types

Code 18 01 01: Sharps, with the exception of sharps from the dialysis treatment of patients who are carriers of blood transmissible viral infections (see reference to code 18 01 03*).
Waste like cannulae, scalpels and objects with similar risks to cause cuts or puncture wounds have to be collected in semisolid and unbreakable disposable containers, securely protected from unauthorised access, as well as transported and disposed of in a secure manner. Joint disposal with non-infectious waste from the dialysis treatment (code 18 01 04) is possible under the view points of epidemic hygiene as long as the issues of occupational health and safety are adhered to.

Code 18 01 02: Body parts and organs including blood bags and blood preservations as long as they do not contain any carriers of transmissible viral infections (reference to code 18 01 03*).
Since in dialysis units this can only mean blood bags and blood preservations which come up only in small quantity, the statement of the LAGA leaflet is limited to individual containers filled with blood or liquid blood products, e.g. a blood preservation which was not used. Their contents can be disposed of into the public sewage system if the occupational health and safety view points in terms of hygiene and prevention of infection are adhered to.

Remark:
In the exceptional case of disposal of complete blood-filled blood lines and dialyser they shall not be emptied but have to be disposed in liquid tight manner.

Code 18 01 03*: Waste whose collection and disposal is subject to special requirements in order to prevent infection.
Special requirements for the collection and disposal of these wastes are only required, if it is expected that the following specified disease can be spread via wastes.

Considered has to be:
- the danger of infection (contagiousness, infective dose, epidemic potential)

- the survivability of the pathogen (length of virulence)
- the path of transmission
- the extent and type of potential contamination
- the quantity of contaminated waste
- the severity of the triggered illness and the possibility of treatment

Remark:
According to the present state of knowledge, waste from this group can arise by the following diseases (listed here are only those infectious diseases which are conceivable in the dialysis units of the geographical region of Germany. Further diseases are listed in the LAGA instruction leaflet).

Disease	**Carrier**	**Path of Transmission**
AIDS/HIV	blood	contact through or via damaged skin or mucosa
HBV, HCV	blood	contact through or via damaged skin or mucosa
TSE (Transmissible spongiform encephalopathy)	tissue, liquor	contact through or via damaged skin or mucosa
CJD, vCJD (Creutzfeldt-Jacob disease)	blood, liquor	contact through or via damaged skin or mucosa
Cholera	faeces, vomit	faecal-oral (smear infection)
Dysentery, HUS (haemolytic uremic syndrome)	faeces	faecal-oral (smear infection)
Typhoid/Paratyphoid fever	faeces, urine, gall, blood	faecal-oral (smear infection)
Active Tuberculosis	sputum, urine, faeces	aerogenous transmission, smear infection
Meningitis/Encephalitis	sputum, pharyngeal secretions	aerogenous transmission, smear infection
Brucellosis	blood	aerogenous transmission, smear infection
Diphtheria	sputum, pharyngeal secretions, wound secretions	aerogenous transmission, smear infection

Detailed knowledge is required for the assessment of risk of infection. Actions within the facility must consider the local circumstances and preconditions in agreement with the infection control specialist, the safety officer and the occupational health specialist.

Concerning infectious diseases e.g. HBV, HCV, HIV, issues of occupational health and safety are a top priority. Correspondingly contaminated sharps, blood-filled vessels, and blood-soaked waste as well as undiluted blood-filled dialysers and blood lines from the treatment of known virus carriers belong to the waste code 18 01 03*. Not included are non-dripping dressings from wounds or operation covers.

The amount of highly blood-contaminated dialysers and blood lines, which has to be disposed of, is small, because the blood of the dialysis patient is always attempted to be rinsed back completely at the end of each treatment if possible.

Sharps, e.g. disposable scalpels, cannulae from the treatment of known virus carriers have to be disposed of either according to the code 18 01 03* as hazardous waste or they have to be decontaminated with the help of thermal procedures.

Code 18 01 04: Waste whose collection and disposal is not subject to special requirements in order to prevent infection.

Apart from the above-described exceptions, all wastes from dialysis units have to be classified under the code 18 01 04 and be jointly disposed of with household waste. Sorting or recycling of these waste materials is forbidden for hygienic reasons. If dialysis wastes are collected by the public waste management service provider together with household waste, the operator of the dialysis facility has to clarify whether the household waste is being brought to a sorting plant. If this is the case, the authority responsible has to be informed. A justified request can be made asking for liberation from the compulsory joint waste disposal and from use of public utilities, this has to be filed and a private disposal company has to be commissioned.

In order to fulfil the high hygienic requirements within the facility,

- waste contaminated with blood, e.g. dressings, blood lines, dialysers, etc., has to be collected and sent off for disposal in tear-proof and fluid-proof containers;
- cannulae and syringes have to be collected in lockable, fluid-proof, puncture-proof and unbreakable disposable containers.

It shall be explicitly pointed out that the waste from the treatment of patients who are colonised by resistant germs, e.g. MRSA or VRE is also to be classified under this fraction of waste. This type of contaminated wastes must be collected in the treatment area in tear- and fluid-proof bags using the double bag method.

Code 18 01 06*: Chemicals Consisting of or Containing Dangerous Substances.

Empty and rinsed-out disinfectant canisters can be collected for recycling. Protective measures for staff have to be respected during the rinsing, good ventilation must be ensured. Before transporting these rinsed containers, any attached notes about hazardous substance must be removed. Drip-free small disinfectant containers can be disposed of through the household waste.

Residues of disinfectant shall not be emptied into the sewage system for disposal purposes. As far as the date of expiry has been exceeded and thus their use according to the regulations is no longer possible, the full or half full containers which have been stored for too long have to be brought to the local pollutants collection. It is advisable to first get in contact with the local waste disposal advisory office. Information given in the safety data sheets about handling of the substance must be adhered to.

10 Examination of the Effectiveness of Disinfection Procedures for Dialysis Machines

Dialysis machines are disinfected and cleaned at different temperature ranges. Thus the effectiveness of the disinfection procedures has to be methodically separated and assessed.

Three procedures are to be distinguished:
- chemical, temperature < 60 °C
- chemo-thermic, temperature > 60 °C, < 90 °C
- thermal, temperature > 90 °C

During the examination of the effectiveness different testing organisms are employed.

Besides suspension tests (laboratory examinations for disinfectants), the examinations also contain practically oriented tests, i.e. procedures which portray a combination of dialyser and product. Purely thermal disinfection is only tested in practical procedures. The germ count reduction must amount to at least 5-log steps in all the testing methods[135].

At the moment, there are no uniform European norms yet for the assessment of disinfection procedures for dialysis machines. The effectiveness has to be proven by the manufacturers within the framework of the medical devices admission procedure. The operator can ask the manufacturer for the corresponding certificates.

[135] Standardmethoden der DGHM zur Prüfung chemischer Desinfektionsverfahren

11 Check Lists and Forms

11.1 Home Haemodialysis – Preconditions and Operation

Requirements for Home Haemodialysis				
Planning/Preparation	**Sections/Subjects**	**Criteria/Requirements**	**Measures/Goals/Controls**	**Remarks**
Structural preconditions	Storeroom for sterile goods	Temperature	5 °C to 25 °C see product information	– No direct solar radiation – No parasites
		Ventilation, humidity	Prevent the formation of mould	
		Entry only for those concerned		
	Treatment room	Floor covering	Fluid-proof, disinfectable partial covering in the dialysis section	
		Hand basin, inlet and outlet, storage areas	Near the treatment	
Water purification	Inspection of the domestic water connection public network/self-supply	Pre-treatment of drinking water according to the instructions of the manufacturer	Water analysis and evaluation by the manufacturer	New Drinking Water Ordinance (TWV) regulates the responsibilities of the operators
		Official approval for water extraction in case of self-supply if necessary	Sampling collection at the extraction site	
		Observe chlorine content	Purification depending on the circumstances	Use carbon filters if necessary
Surroundings	General domestic hygiene	Hand disinfectant dispenser		
	Pets/potted plants	Not in the treatment section		Applies for HD and PD
Disposal	Consumables	Disposal routes, no access for other occupants/children	Locking of rooms and blocking pathways (if necessary)	Frequent emptying and/or separate containers if necessary

Running Operation				
Water purification after consultation and suggestion of the manufacturer due analyses of the supply water	Pre-treatment depending on circumstances and analyses	Control scheme	Regular controls	Regular information of the water supplier desired
	Domestic water entrance filter	Pollution level and pressure drop	Regular controls and change (min. 1/year or difference > 0.5 bar)	Maintenance according to the manufacturer
	Softener as required	Product information	Regeneration before the start of treatment	Maintenance according to the manufacturer
	Reverse osmosis	Preventive measures	At least 1 rinsing cycle on treatment-free days	Product information
		Routine disinfection in accordance with product information	e.g. disinfection procedures 1/month Remark: Higher frequency might be necessary if microbiological results are out of specification	When time of non-use is greater > 3 days or in accordance with the product information
Dialyser	Permeate inflow	Preventive measures	Change min. 1/year and afterwards microbiological examination of the permeate	Desirable: inclusion of the permeate inflow in the disinfection cycle
	Ultrafilter ("Sterile filter")	Preventive measures	Change according to product information	
Dialyser	Dialysate outflow		Free outlet (DIN 1988 (EN 1717))	
	Hydraulics	Disinfection	According to product information	Before and after the treatment
		Cleaning	According to product information	Influencing factors: dialyser and the patients' lipid metabolism
	Surfaces	Cleaning and Disinfection	After every treatment	
Patient	Personal hygiene	Skin and hand hygiene	Education plan e.g. – Technique and surroundings – Treatment with/without partner – Hygiene and disinfection – Self-observation and care – Handling of biological waste	See basic rules for the prevention of infections
	Special hygiene	Shunt hygiene		
				Further education if required
	Handling sterile goods			DIN 58953 Part 8 Supply of Sterile Goods
	Handling of hazardous substances	Guidelines for the household		Operating instructions
	Disposal of medical wastes			Observe communal statutes
Medications	Medication or drugs requiring cooling	Storage	Refrigerator (closed box)	Use in accordance with the product information
	Other medications	Storage	Light proof at room temperature	

11.2 Peritoneal Dialysis – Preconditions and Operation

Requirements for CAPD = Continuous Ambulatory Peritoneal Dialysis APD = Automated Peritoneal Dialysis				
Planning/Preparation	**Sections**	**Criteria/Requirements**	**Measures/Goals/Controls**	**Remarks**
Structural Precondi-tions	Store room for sterile goods	Temperature	5 °C to 25 °C see product information	– No direct solar radiation – No parasites
		Ventilation, humidity	Prevent the formation of mould	
		Entry only for those concerned		
	Treatment room	Floor covering	Fluid-proof, disinfectable partial covering of the dialysis section	
		Hand basin, outlet, storage areas		
Surroundings	General household hygiene	Hand disinfectant dispenser		
	Pets, plants	Not in the treatment section		
Disposal	Consumables	Disposal pathways, no access for other occupants/children	Locking of rooms and blocking pathways (if necessary)	Frequent emptying and/or separate containers (if necessary)
Running Operation				
Cycler	Dialysate outflow		Free outlet	
	Surfaces	Cleaning	After every treatment	

Patient	Personal hygiene	Skin and hand hygiene	Education plan e.g. – Technique and surroundings – Treatment with/without partner – Hygiene and disinfection – Self-observation and care – Handling biological waste	Basic rules for the prevention of infections
		Catheter hygiene		
		Changing of PD bag		Further education if required
		Aseptic working technique		
	Handling sterile goods			DIN 58953 Part 8 Supply of Sterile Goods
	Dealing with hazardous substances			Operating instructions
	Disposal of medical wastes			Observe communal statutes/empty pouches non-recyclable material
	Dealing with biological waste	If possible no handling		CES/peritonitis infection
Medications	Medication or drugs requiring cooling	Storage	Refrigerator (closed box)	Use in accordance with Product information
	Other medications	Storage	Light proof at room temperature	

11.3 Quality Requirements for Drinking Water and Permeate

	Drinking water [mg/l = ppm]	Permeate [mg/l = ppm		
	Drinking Water Ordinance: Amendment of 21.05.2001 (Extract)	AAMI RD 62 (2001)	Ph. Eur. 5.0 (Europ. Pharmacopoeia) 01/2005:1167	Recommendation of the guideline of the hygiene working group
Sodium (Na)	200	70	50	50
Potassium (K)	–.–	8	2	8
Calcium (Ca)	–.–	2	2	2
Magnesium (Mg)	–.–	4	2	4
Barium (B)	1	–.–	–.–	–.–
Barium (Ba)	–.–	0.1	–.–	0.1
Ammonium (NH4)	0.5	–.–	0.2	0.2
Aluminium (Al)	0.2	0.01	0.01	0.01
Heavy metal			0.1	
– Copper (Cu)	2	0.1		0.1
– Arsenic (As)	0.01	0.005		0.005
– Lead (Pb)	0.01	0.005		0.005
– Silver (Ag)	–.–	0.005		0.005
– Chromium (Cr)	0.05	0.014		0.014
– Selenium (Se)	0.01	0.09		0.01
– Antimony (Sb)	0.005	0.006		0.005
– Mercury (Hg)	0.001	0.002	0.001	0.0002
– Nickel (Ni)	0.02	–.–		–.–
– Stannum (Sn)	–.–	–.–		–.–
– Iron (Fe)	0.2	–.–		–.–
– Cadmium (Cd)	0.005	0.001		0.001
– Zinc (Zn)	–.–	0.1	0.1	0.1
– Manganese (Mn)	0.05			

Cyanide (CN)	0.05	0.02	-.–	0.02
Chlorine (Cl_2)	–.–	0.5	0.1	0.1
Chloride (Cl)	250	–.–	50	50
Chloramine	–.–	0.1	-.–	0.1
Fluoride (F)	1.5	0.2	0.2	0.2
Sulphate (SO_4)	240	100	50	50
Nitrate (NO_3)	50	2	2	2
Nitrite (NO_2)	0.1	–.–	–.–	–.–
Organic Chlorine compounds	0.05	0.1	–.–	0.1
Polycyclic aromatic hydrocarbons	0.0001	–.–	–.–	–.–
pH	6.5 – 9.5	–.–	–.–	–.–
Conductivity	2500 µS/cm at 20 °C	–.–	–.–	–.–
Bacteriology [cfu/ml]	< 100 (22 °C) < 20 (36 °C)	< 200 (35-37 °C, 48 hrs)	< 100 (30-35 °C, 5 days)	< 100 according to RKI (22 ± 2 °C, 3-7 days)
Pyrogenicity	–.–	< 2 EU/ml =	< 0.25 IU/ml	< 0.25 IU/ml

Remark:
In the Drinking Water Ordinance and the AAMI, critical values for rare substances which have not been listed here can be looked up in the original publications. In comparison to previous publications of the Drinking Water Ordinance, the AAMI and the European Pharmacopoeia, no details are given about nitrogen and phosphate.
In comparison tc the previous guideline, the critical values found in the guidelines of the European Council of the EC and the DIN drafts of 1987 have been taken out. The amended Drinking Water Ordinance implements the critical values of the European Council; a new DIN draft is not known.

11.4 Letter to Communal Water Suppliers

To the
[Communal Water Supplier]
....
....
[Place], [Date]

Dear Madam/Sir,

The artificial kidney places high requirements on the quality of water used. For your information, I have included a copy of the present quality standards for "water used in diluting concentrated haemodialysis solutions". If these quality standards are not fulfilled, this can lead to life-threatening situations for the patient.
Chemicals like aluminium, fluoride, free chlorine and chloramine especially those which are generally used in purifying communal water can seriously affect the health of haemodialysis patients.
We have installed a water purification plant in our dialysis centre which under normal circumstances enables us to arrive at the required quality standard needed for water used in diluting concentrated haemodialysis solutions. This water purification system was specially designed and put together based on the average composition of the water you supply.
The plant consists of (an active carbon filter), a water softener as well as a reverse osmosis unit. These components are capable of removing all the substances found in the drinking water which could be harmful to the patient.
We would like to kindly ask you to inform us immediately of every change in the water composition especially the use of disinfectants like chlorine, or the dosing of other chemicals so that we can order the corresponding measures needed for the protection of our patients.

Thank you very much for your understanding and collaboration.

Yours sincerely,

11.5 Return of Dialysis Machines from Patients with Blood-Transmissible Viral Infections

Protocol-Form

Proof of disinfection for the return of a machine from an infectious to a non-infectious section.

Reprocessing according to the guidelines of applied hygiene in dialysis treatment units.
(The instructions for use and the 10 testing methods for disinfection shall be observed for the performance!)

Dialyser, Type and No. ______________________
Last Location: ______________________
Section: ______________________
Responsible for the realisation of the disinfection (Name): __________
Head or Responsible Physician of the Dialysis Treatment Unit (Name): ______________________

1. Machine Disinfection + Decalcification, Date: __________

Disinfectant: ______________________
Procedure: ______________________

2. Machine Disinfection + Cleaning, Date: __________

Disinfectant: ______________________
Procedure: ______________________

Surface Disinfection

Disinfectant: ______________________
Concentration: ______________________
Effective exposure time: ______________________ (min.)

Date:	Date:
Physician:	Responsible for the Performance of the Disinfection
(Signature)	(Signature)

11.6 HBV Diagnostics[136]

Examination	Examined Parameters	Test Results	Interpretation
Initial Examination:	**HBsAg + Anti-HBc + Anti-HBs**	No positive marker:	• Not infected • Not immune
		HBsAg + Anti-HBc-positive:	• Existing infection
		Anti-HBs + Anti-HBc-positive:	• Immunity after infection
		Only HBsAg-positive:	• HBV infected • Additional test
		Only anti-HBs-positive:	• Immunity
		Only Anti-HBc:	• Possibly HBV infected • Immunity not guaranteed • HBV-Vaccination (if necessary) • Additional test
Confirmatory test if HBsAg-positive (facultative)	**HBsAg**	HBsAg-positive:	• HBV-infected
		HBsAg-negative:	• Not infected • Not immune • (false-positive HBsAg-Test)
Additional test: if Anti-HBc isolated positive	**HBV-DNA**	HBV-DNA-positive:	• HBV-infected
		HBV-DNA-negative:	• Immunity uncertain • HBV vaccination

136 www.kompetenznetz-hepatitis.de/aerzteforum/hep_net/diagnostik.htm

Control examinations:	**HBsAg + Anti-HBc**	No positive marker:	• Not infected
Additional test: If HBsAg and/or Anti-HBc first time positive:	**Anti-HBc IgM**	Anti-HBc-IgM-positive:	• Fresh HBV infection
		Anti-HBc-IgM-negative:	For confirmed HBsAg: • Previous HBV infection
Additional test: Only when Anti-HBc first time positive	**HBV-DNA**	HBV-DNA-positive:	• HBV infection
		HBV-DNA-negative:	• False-positive Anti-HBc test? • Previous infection?
Controls	**Anti-HBs**	After vaccination	Pos. > 100 IU/l control after 12 months Pos. > 50 IU/l control after 6 months Pos. < 10 - 50 IU/l revaccinate neg. after > 5 vaccinations = Non-Responder
Screening for risk factors (e.g. holiday dialysis, transfusions)	**Transaminase GOT and GPT**		If value is increased: HBV Serology Test

11.7 HCV Diagnostics[137]

Examination	Examined Parameters	Test Results	Interpretation
Initial Examination:	**Anti-HCV + HCV-RNA**	No positive marker:	• Not infected
		Only HCV-RN-positive:	• HCV infected
		Only Anti-HCV-positive	• HCV contact, previous HCV • Further HCV-RNA confirmatory test
		Anti-HCV + HCV-RNA-positive	• HCV infected
Confirmatory test only when Anti-HCV-positive	**HCV-RNA**	HCV-RNA-negative:	• Not infected (false-positive Anti-HCV test)
		HCV-RNA-positive:	• Existing infection
		HCV-RNA-positive from previous test results, then the tests must be three times negative within one year	• Probably previous HCV infection (?)
Control examination	**Anti-HCV**	Anti-HCV-negative	• Not infected
		Anti-HCV-positive	• Confirmatory test RIBA or immediate HCV-RNA test
Confirmatory test only when Anti-HCV-positive with or without an available positive HCV-RNA test	**RIBA (Immunoblot-antibody confirmatory test)**	Anti-HCV immuno-blot-negative	• Not infected (false-positive anti-HCV test)
		Anti-HCV Immunoblot-positive	• Continue with HCV-RNA test
Screening for risk factors (e.g. holiday dialysis, transfusions)	**Transaminase**	GOT and GPT	Already a slight increase may indicate a contamination or infection, further diagnostic clarification is necessary

137 www.kompetenznetz-hepatitis.de/aerzteforum/hep_net/diagnostik.htm

11.8 Post Exposure Prophylaxis (PEP) for Staff

Emergency measures – as documented in the hygiene plan

Stab or cut wound

Increase blood flow by administering pressure/ Encourage blood flow through pressure on the surrounding tissue (> 1 minute)

Contamination of damaged skin, eye or oral cavity

Intensive rinsing with the nearest accessible: high-proof (denatured for the oral cavity) alcohol, water or isotone sodium chloride solution, PVP-iodine solution[1] (if necessary)

Intensive antiseptic rinsing or application/ laying of an antiseptic agent depot[1]

Systemic medicamentous post exposure prophylaxis if necessary

Documentation of Accident (Contact accident insurance consultant or physician)

First HIV antibody test, hepatitis serology

[1] For the skin: alcohol-based skin antiseptic
for wounds: > 80% ethanol-based preparations (e.g. Frekaderm)
or high-proof alcohol-based preparation + PVP-iodine (e.g. Betaseptic)
For the eyes: e.g. isotone watery PVP-iodine solution 2.5%

11.9 Indication for the Initiation of Pharmacotherapy as Post Exposure Prophylaxis (PEP) in Case of Exposure to HIV

Contact with HIV-positive blood through percutaneous injury,e.g. injection needles	Recommended
Contact to mucosa or injured/damaged skin with fluids containing high concentrations of viruses, e.g. blood	Offer
Percutaneous contact, skin contact and mucosa contact with body fluids like urine and saliva	Not recommended
Contact of intact skin with blood, also in case of high virus concentration	Not recommended

138, 139

11.10 HBV Post Exposure Prophylaxis (PEP) for Staff after Presumable Contact with HBV-Containing Material

No immuno-prophylaxis necessary:

- If less than 5 years have elapsed since a successful basic immunisation for HBV (Anti-HBs > 100 IU/l).
- If within the last 12 months, an Anti-HBs concentration of > 100 IU/l was proven.

Immediate administration of a single HBV booster injection:

- If a successful basic immunisation (Anti-HBs > 100 IU/l) was carried out 5-10 years ago.

The immediate testing of the exposed persons for Anti-HBs has to take place:

- If the last HBV vaccination took place more than 10 years ago.

[138] Empfehlungen zur HIV-Postexpositionsprophylaxe (www.rki.de)

[139] Postexpositionelle Prophylaxe der HIV-Exposition/PEP, Deutsch-Österreichische Empfehlung (www.rki.de)

- If no vaccination was done or the vaccination was incomplete.
- If after the basic immunisation < 100 IU/l Anti-HBs were measured (low or Non-Responder).
- If the success of the vaccination after the HBV vaccination was not confirmed using a quantitative Anti-HBs test.

Procedure after Test Results:

Test Results:	Necessary Measures:
In case of confirmation of > 100 IU/l:	No immuno-prophylaxis necessary
In case of confirmation of 10-100 IU/l:	Administration of a single HBV booster injection
In case of < 10 IU/l or impossibility of testing within 48 hours:	Administration of hepatitis B immuno-globulin and beginning or completion of a hepatitis B vaccination

140

11.11 HCV Post Exposure Prophylaxis (PEP) for Staff

After a presumable contact with HCV-containing material, the following measures have to be undertaken in addition to the conservative post exposure prophylaxis:

1. Determination of the HCV antibodies: immediately, after 6 weeks and after 6 months
2. Determination of the transaminase: immediately, after 6 weeks and after 6 months
3. Determination of the HCV-RNA with PCR: after 2 weeks and 6 weeks

If the HCV-RNA is positive, an antiviral therapy with PEG Interferon and Ribavin has to be tried.

[140] Recommendations of the Permanent Vaccination Commission (STIKO) at the Robert Koch Institute/State: July 2004. Epidemiological Bulletin 23rd July 2004 (30): 235-250

11.12 Hygiene Measures during Infectious Illnesses

Measures	Blood Transmissible Viral Infections			Methicillin-resistant Staphylococcus aureus		Tuberculosis (Tb)		Infectious Gastroenteritis	
Notification requirement according to the Infections Protection Act (IfSG §..)	**By name, suspicion, illness and death (§ 6)**		**Not by name, the direct and indirect evidence (§ 7 sect. 3)**	**Not by name, the frequent occurrence like nosocomial infection as outbreak (§ 6 sect. 3)**		**by name, persons affected with therapy-requiring Tb, or death due to (confirmed) (§ 6)**		**By name, suspicion and illness in case of frequent occurrences in epidemic context (§ 6 clause 2b)**	
	HBV	HCV	HIV	nose-pharynx, skin	wound, dry dressing	suspicion	open	Norovirus	remaining
Spatial Assignment									
Separate unit	–	–	–	❶	–	–	●	–	–
Separate room/zones	❶	❶	●	❷	–	●	–	●	–
Functional isolation	–	❷	–	–		–		❷	❶
Own dialysis machine	●	●	●	–		–	●	–	–
Scrub/wet disinfection	●		●	●		●	*●	*●	●
Crockery									
Disinfectable dishwasher	❶		❶	❶	❶	❶		❶	
Transport box for dirty crockery	–		–		–			–	
Disposable crockery	❷		❷	❷	❷	❷		❷	
Staff									
Protective overall (infection specific to patient groups)	●	●	●	●		●		●	●
Wearing a mask for every contact with patients	–		–	●	O Change of dressing	●	● FFP 2	●	–
Head cap	–		–	–		–		–	–
Gloves	●		●	●		●		●	
Disinfection of hands	●		●	●		● observe product information		● product information	●
Protective glasses	Eye or face protection, if splashing or spraying of infectious or potentially infectious materials or fluids is to be expected.								

● necessary O recommended ❶ best solution ❷ possible alternative * substance and concentration according to RKI

Measures	Blood Transmissible Viral Infections			Methicillin-resistant Staphylococcus aureus		Tuberculosis (Tb)		Infectious Gastroenteritis	
Notification requirement according to the Infections Protection Act (IfSG §..)	**By name, suspicion, illness and death (§ 6)**		**Not by name, the direct and indirect evidence (§ 7 sect. 3)**	**Not by name, the frequent occurrence like nosocomial infection as outbreak (§ 6 sect. 3)**		**by name, persons affected with therapy-requiring Tb, or death due to (confirmed) (§ 6)**		**By name, suspicion and illness in case of frequent occurrences in epidemic context (§ 6 clause 2b)**	
	HBV	HCV	HIV	nose-pharynx, skin	wound, dry dressing	suspicion	open	Norovirus	remaining
Patient									
Patient-related material	●	●	●	● Disposing of openly stored material	–	●		●	●
Own RR-machine/tourniquet	●	●	●	●		●	●	●	–
Hand disinfection (Patient/ Staff) upon entering the facility	–		–	●		●		●	
Before leaving the room	●		○	●		●		●	
Gloves for shunt compression	●		●	●		○		○	
Wearing a mask and protective overall before entering and when leaving	–		–	●	–	●		–	–
Own toilet	–		–	○	–	●		❶ [141]	
Transport of inf. pat./ ambulance	–		–	● register	–	● register		●	–
Separate transport/taxi				●	–	●		●	–

● necessary ○ recommended ❶ best solution ❷ possible alternative * substance and concentration according to RKI

141 Disinfection necessary after every patient

Measures	Blood Transmissible Viral Infections			Methicillin-resistant Staphylococcus aureus		Tuberculosis (Tb)		Infectious Gastroenteritis	
Notification requirement according to the Infections Protection Act (IfSG §..)	**By name, suspicion, illness and death (§ 6)**		**Not by name, the direct and indirect evidence (§ 7 sect. 3)**	**Not by name, the frequent occurrence like nosocomial infection as outbreak (§ 6 sect. 3)**		**by name, persons affected with therapy-requiring Tb, or death due to (confirmed) (§ 6)**		**By name, suspicion and illness in case of frequent occurrences in epidemic context (§ 6 clause 2b)**	
	HBV	HCV	HIV	nose-pharynx, skin	wound, dry dressing	suspicion	open	Norovirus	remaining
Disposal	No press-container, not for sharp objects as well								
B waste	●		●	● double bag		–		●	
C waste	● only cannulae / sharps		● only cannulae / sharps	–		●		–	
Laundry/Cleaning									
Disinfectant reprocessing	●		●	● incl. covers and pillows		● incl. covers and pillows		●	
Protected transport	–		–	●		●		●	–
Last room to be cleaned or separate cleaning trolley	○		○	●	–	●		●	–

● necessary ○ recommended ❶ best solution ❷ possible alternative * substance and concentration according to RKI

11.13 Information Sheet for MRSA Patients

Name of Patient: ______________________ Date: __________

You were diagnosed as being colonised with a bacterium called the Methicillin-resistant Staphylococcus aureus (MRSA). The living of the bacteria on your skin, colonisation itself with this bacterium poses no problem to you and does not increase the potential danger for people with intact immuno-reactions.

There is, however, the danger that the bacteria move from your skin or mucosa into a wound and thus get inside your body. For severely immuno-deficient persons like dialysis patients for example, there is an increased danger of transmission with the risk of infection.

For these reasons, we would like to call on you to observe the following instructions:

- If need be, we might call on you to put on a mask for mouth protection (if there is proof of MRSA in the nose or respiratory tract) and disinfect your hands before entering the dialysis centre. The mask has to be worn until you have settled onto your dialysis bed. At the end of the dialysis and before leaving the bed, the mask has to be put on again and it has to be taken off only after leaving the dialysis centre.
- Upon entering the dialysis centre, you first have to carefully disinfect your hands with the corresponding disinfectant solution. Only after this is it possible to go to the toilet for example. In principle, please avoid touching surfaces and objects and rather ask the nurses for help instead. Careful disinfection of the hands is also necessary after using the toilet. After using the toilet, please carry out a spray disinfection of the toilet seat with an alcoholic surface disinfection spray. Let the staff hand-over a bottle with alcoholic surface disinfection spray to you. You shall also carefully treat your hands again with hand

disinfectant at the end of the treatment and before leaving the dialysis centre.

- You shall apply Turixin ointment in every nostril 3 to 5 times per day for at least 5 days (the quantity shall be about one match head big pushed into each nostril using a cotton bud). Then press the nose together and massage it afterwards between the thumb and index finger. A disinfection of the hands must be carried out at the end.
- You have to properly gurgle with Polyhexanide-containing gargle e.g. PRONTOSAN® solution (1:1 diluted with tea) three times a day for at least 5 days.
- In the same way, you have to take a medicated tub bath, be washed in bed or do a shower washing (incl. hair and head) for at least 5 days every day.

Bath:
Here the whole body including the hair is bathed for about 20 minutes in bath water prepared with 4-times SANALIND® (800 ml in ca. 80 l water) for example. Add an additional washing lotion like FREKA® MED on the flannel mitt.

Washing in bed:
Warm washing-water solution with 4-times SANALIND® (1 l for 3 l water) shall be prepared. Additionally add FREKA® MED washing lotion on a flannel mitt; wash off with Sanalind washing-water.

Shower washing:
Shower off with warm water, lather with undiluted FREKA® MED soap lotion, leave on for 3 minutes to take effect, shower off with warm water, then repeat again.

Afterwards, the sections of the external auricle and the external auditory canal are rubbed in using FREKA® MED-soaked fresh cotton buds. Fresh underwear and clothes shall be worn daily after bathing or showering; a fresh towel shall be used every day. In the same way too, the bed linen has to be changed daily for at least 5 days. The changed clothes, towels and bed linen have to be washed using a thermal (80-90 °C) or chemo-thermal laundry procedure. Paper tissues shall be used as handkerchiefs. These are to be disposed of after single use.

- The success of these measures will be regularly controlled by means of swab examinations. At the end of the decontamination measures – normally after at least 5 days but often up to 10 days for dialysis patients – a decontamination-free interval of 2 days remains. Afterwards, swabs will be carried out on three successive dialysis days (first swab after > 24 hrs and < 48 hrs). The sustained success will be controlled again after 30 days and after 3 months as long as there has been no proof of MRSA on the swabs taken directly after the measures. If a control swab is positive, the decontamination will be continued and controls carried out as previously described.
- It has to be emphasised once more that the MRSA bacterium poses no danger for healthy persons in ambulatory and domestic sections. Only contact persons with open wounds or skin rashes are at risk of getting infected with MRSA. Physical contact shall be avoided with these persons during the time that they are MRSA-carriers.
- Persons in your surroundings (family, old or nursing homes) shall be made aware of the content of this information letter. If necessary, we will also get in contact with these persons to discuss the above-mentioned measures.

Date: ____________ Physician's Signature: ____________________

I have been fully explained the above-mentioned information and I fully understand it. I will implement the prescribed measures as discussed.

Date: ____________ Patient's Signature ______________________

11.14 MRSA Infection – Plan for procedure – EXAMPLE[142]

Measures	Date/ Abbr.
1. Risk patient defined: ☐ chronic wound ☐ MRSA in the anamnesis ☐ comes from institution with frequent cases of MRSA ☐ swabs carried out	
2. Swab results incl. antibiotic resistance program from the lab seen. MRSA diagnosis is available.	
3. Carrying out of swabs on further preferred localisation if necessary; (hairline, ears, both vestibules of the nose, pharynx, both axillae, both sides of the groin)	
4. The dialysis for the affected person will be carried out till further notice in room ______________ or a so-called functional isolation will take place in accordance with the hygiene plan. In each case and independent of where the dialysis treatment takes place, think also of hand disinfection after every contact with the patient and remind all the colleagues once more!	
5. Education information of the patient and making contact with ☐ Family physician ☐ Ambulance service company ☐ Relatives and/or homecare or nursing home support ☐ Kitchen (disposable crockery or sealed transportation of crockery) ☐ Housekeeping (laundry)	
6. ☐ Give information sheet to the patients and relatives/ nursing home	
7. Due to the situation and the general condition of the patient, the decontamination measures will be carried out over a period of 5-10 days as ☐ Bath – preparation/prescription given to take along ☐ Shower washing – preparation/prescription given to take along ☐ Washing in bed – preparation/prescription given to take along	

[142] Zastrow et al: Concept for the Decontamination of MRSA Patients Hyg Med 2001 (26): 344-348

Measures	Date/ Abbr.
7.1 For bath or washing in bed, issue prescription to the patient for: a) MUPIROCIN ointment – 3 gr. (e.g. TURIXIN®) b) POLYHEXANID gargle – 500 ml (e.g. PRONTOSAN® D) c) POLYHEXANID-washing lotion – 10 x 1000 ml (e.g. FREKA® MED) d) POLYHEXANID-bath preparation 6 x 2 litres (e.g. SANALIND® 4-times)	
7.2. For shower washing issue prescription to the patient for: a) MUPIROCIN ointment – 3 gr. (e.g. TURIXIN®) b) POLYHEXANIDE gargle – 500 ml (e.g. PRONTOSAN® D) c) POLYHEXANIDE washing lotion – 10 x 1000 ml (e.g. FREKA® MED)	
8. For the treatment of wounds, issue prescription to the patient for: a) POLYHEXANIDE concentrate – 5 x 2 ml (e.g. LAVASEPT®) b) SODIUM CHLORIDE SOLUTION 0.9% – 5 x 500 ml from dialysis stock c) THREAD-BOTTLE – 1 ml Lavasept® in 500 ml NaCl for 0.2% solution	
The additional note "MRSA therapy" on the prescription is useful as a justification to the health insurance institution.	
9. Instructing the patient or family and nursing home if necessary on Hand disinfection Wearing mouth protection mask Using Turixin (Mupirocin) ointment Gurgling Showering and washing procedure Bathing sequence Changing linen and laundry Duration of use	
10. Swab control of preferred localisation and the wound if necessary on the 3rd, 4th and 5th day after the end of the decontamination measures, or three times on successive dialysis (like in 4.).	
11. Calling off the isolation measures if the controls are negative thrice.	

Physician's Signature: Signature of the responsible nurse:

11.15 Template for Catering

Calendar week		Monday	Tuesday	Wednesday	Thursday	Friday	Saturday	Corrective Measure
Income goods Control (Delivery through caterer, wholesale market, large kitchen)								
Shrink-wrapped sausage < 7 °C BBD	Temperature							
	BBD							
	Initials							
Shrink-wrapped cheese < 7 °C BBD	Temperature							
	BBD							
	Initials							
Fresh sausage < 7 °C	Temperature							
	Initials							
Filled rolls (sausage/cheese) < 7 °C	Temperature							
	Initials							
Frozen meals < –18 °C	Temperature							
	Initials							
Warm delivered meals > 65 °C	Temperature							
	Initials							
Cold delivered meals to be heated up (small sausages, meatballs) < 7 °C	Temperature							
	Initials							
Cleaning state of the container used for transport	OK							
	Initials							
Disinfection of the foodstuff thermometer after utilisation	Carried out							
	Initials							

BBD = Best-before date
How often controls of incoming goods are to be carried out has to be codified in the hygiene plan.

Calendar week		**Monday**	**Tuesday**	**Wednesday**	**Thursday**	**Friday**	**Saturday**	**Corrective Measure**
Storage Controls/every working day								
Foodstuff refrigerator I < 7 °C	Temperature							
	Staff Initials							
Foodstuff refrigerator II < 7 °C	Temperature							
	Initials							
Foodstuff refrigerator III < 7 °C	Temperature							
	Initials							
Freezer I < –18 °C	Temperature							
	Initials							
Freezer II < –18 °C	Temperature							
	Initials							
Freezer III < –18 °C	Temperature							
	Initials							
Distribution Controls/at least 1/week								
Frozen meals > 65 °C	Temperature							
	Initials							
Warm delivered meals > 65 °C	Temperature							
	Initials							
Self-heated meals (sausages, meatballs) > 65 °C	Temperature							
	Initials							
Disinfection of the foodstuff thermometer after utilisation	Carried out							
	Initials							

Calendar week		Monday	Tuesday	Wednesday	Thursday	Friday	Saturday	Corrective Measure
Incoming goods Control (Proof for the observance of the cold chain in case of self-purchase)								
Shrink-wrapped sausage and/or meat products < 7 °C BBD	Temp. in the cold box							
	BBD							
	Initials							
Shrink-wrapped cheese < 7 °C BBD	Temp. in the cold box							
	BBD							
	Initials							
Fresh sausage and/or fresh cheese < 7 °C	Temp. in the cold box							
	Initials							
Frozen foods < –18°C	Temp. in the deep-freeze box							
	BBD							
	Initials							
Cleaning state of the cold box and the cooling or deep-freeze container	OK							
	Initials							
Disinfection of the thermometer	Carried out							
	Initials							

BBD = Best-before date

The stock receipt control has to be carried out and documented for every purchase.

12 Abbreviations

Abbreviation/ Term	Explanation in German	Explanation in English
A		
AAMI	Association for the Advancement of Medical Instrumentation	Association for the Advancement of Medical Instrumentation
AbfG	Abfallgesetz	Waste Disposal Law
AfnP	Arbeitsgemeinschaft für nephrologisches Pflegepersonal	Working Group of Nephrological Nursing Staff (PO)
AMG	Arzneimittelgesetz	German Pharmaceutical Act
ArbSchG	Arbeitsschutzgesetz	Industrial Safety Act
AS	Abfallschlüssel	Waste Code
AV-Fistel	Arterio-venöse Fistel	Arteriovenous shunt or fistula
AVV	Abfallverzeichnis-verordnung	Waste Catalogue Ordinance
B		
BGB	Bürgerliches Gesetzbuch	German Civil Code
BGR	Berufsgenossenschaft-liche Regeln	Regulations of Employers Liability Insurance Association
BGV	Berufsgenossenschaft-liche Vorschriften	Regulations of the Employers' Liability Insurance Association
BgVV	Bundesinstitut für gesundheitlichen Verbraucherschutz und Veterinärmedizin	Federal Institute for Health Protection of Consumers and Veterinary Medicine

BioStoffV	Biostoffverordnung	Biological Agents Ordinance
C		
CEN	Comité Européen de Normalisation	European Committee for Standardisation
CJK	Creutzfeldt-Jakob-Krankheit	Creutzfeldt-Jacob disease
D		
DAGKN	Deutsche Arbeitsgemeinschaft für klinische Nephrologie	German Working Group for Clinical Nephrology (PO)
DGHM	Deutsche Gesellschaft für Hygiene und Mikrobiologie	German Society for Hygiene and Microbiology (PO)
DGKH	Deutsche Gesellschaft für Krankenhaushygiene	German Association of Hospital Hygiene (PO)
DIN	Deutsches Institut für Normung e.V.	German Institute for Standardisation
DKE	Deutsche Kommission Elektrotechnik, Elektronik	German Commission for Electrical, Electronic & Information Technologies
DKG	Deutsche Krankenhausgesellschaft	Association of German Hospitals (PO)
DNA (DNS)	Desoxyribonukleinsäure	Deoxyribonucleic acid
DOQI	Dialysis Outcome Quality Initiative	Dialysis Outcome Quality Initiative
DVG	Deutsche Veterinärmedizinische Gesellschaft	German Society for Veterinary Medicine (PO)
DVV	Deutsche Gesellschaft zur Bekämpfung von Viruskrankheiten	German Association against Virus Diseases

E		
EDTNA/ERCA	European Dialysis and Transplant Nurses Association/European Renal Care Association	European Dialysis and Transplant Nurses Association/European Renal Care Association (PO)
EN	Europäische Norm	European Standard
EU	Europäische Union	European Union
Europharm	Europäische Pharmakopoe	European Pharmacopoeia
EWG	Europäische Wirtschaftsgemeinschaft	European Economic Community (EEC)
F		
FnB	Fachverband für Nephrologische Berufsgruppen	Organisation for Renal Professional Groups
G		
GefstoffV	Gefahrstoffverordnung	Ordinance on Hazardous Substances
GewO	Gewerbeordnung	Industrial Code
GML	Gesellschaft für Medizintechnik und Logistikmanagement	Association for Medical Engineering and Logistics Management (PO)
GOT	Glutamat-Oxalazetat-Transaminase	Glutamic-oxalacetic transaminase
GPT	Glutamat-Pyruvat-Transaminase	Glutamic-pyruvic transaminase
H		
HACCP	Hazard Analysis and Critical Control Points	Hazard Analysis and Critical Control Points
HAV	Hepatitis-A-Virus	Hepatitis A Virus
HBc	Hepatitis B-core	Hepatitis B-core
HBsAg	Hepatitis B-Surface-Antigen	Hepatitis B-Surface-Antigen

HBV	Hepatitis-B-Viren	Hepatitis B Virus
HCV	Hepatitis-C-Viren	Hepatitis C Virus
HD	Hämodialyse	Haemodialysis
HDF	Hämodiafiltration	Haemodiafiltration
HD-PE-Rohre	High Density-Polyethylen-Rohre	High Density Polyethylene Pipes
Hep B	Hepatitis B	Hepatitis B
Hep C	Hepatitis C	Hepatitis C
HF	Hämofiltration	Haemofiltration
HGB	Handelsgesetzbuch	Commercial Code
HGV	Hepatitis-G-Virus	Hepatitis G Virus
HIV	Human Immuno-deficiency Virus	Human Immuno-deficiency Virus
I		
IfSG	Infektionsschutz-gesetz	Infections Protection Act
Ifw	Institut für Fort- und Weiterbildung	Institute for Vocational and Further Training (Education)
IgM	Immunglobulin M	Immunoglobulin M
IPD	Intermittierende Peritonealdialyse	Intermittent Peritoneal Dialysis
IU/L	Internationale Einheit (IE)/Liter	International Unit/Litre
K		
KAST	Katheteraustrittsstelle	Catheter Exit Site
KBE	Koloniebildende Einheiten	colony-forming units (cfu)
KrW	Kreislaufwirtschaft	Closed Substance Cycle Waste Management
L		
LAGA	Länderarbeitsgemein-schaft Abfall	State Working Group "Waste"

LMBG	Lebensmittel- und Bedarfsgegenstände-gesetz	Foodstuffs and Consumer Goods Law
LMHV	Lebensmittelhygiene-verordnung	Foodstuffs Hygiene Ordinance
M		
MDD	EU-Richtlinie über Medizinprodukte	Medical Device Directive
MHD	Mindesthaltbarkeits-datum	Best-before date (BBD)
MP	Medizinprodukt	Medical device
MPBetreibV	Medizinprodukte-Betreiberverordnung	Medical Device Operator Ordinance
MPG	Medizinprodukt-gesetz	Medical Products Act
MRE	Multiresistente Erreger	Multi-resistant pathogens
MRSA	Methicillin-resistenter Staphylococcus aureus	Methicillin (multiple) resistant Staphylo-coccus aureus
N		
NachwV	Nachweisverordnung	Law of Proof of Substantial Conditions Applicable to the Em-ployment Relationship
NKF US	National Kidney Foun-dation US	National Kidney Foundation US
O		
OP	Operation	Operation
OwiG	Ordnungswidrig-keitengesetz	Regulatory Offences Act
P		
PCR	Polymerase Kettenreaktion	Polymerase Chain Reaction
PD	Peritonealdialyse	Peritoneal Dialysis

PDCA	Plan – Do – Check – Act	Plan – Do – Check – Act
PEP	Postexpositionelle Prophylaxe	Post Exposure Prophylaxis
Ph.Eur.	Europäische Pharmakopoe	European Pharmacopoeia
PHV	Der Dialysepartner Patienten-Heimversorgung gemeinnützige Stiftung	The Dialysis Partner of the Patient's Homecare Association (PO)
Q		
QM	Qualitätsmanagement	Quality Management
Quasi Niere	Qualitätssicherung Niere	Organisation "Quality Assurance Kidney"
R		
RDA	Reinigungs- und Desinfektionsanlage	Cleaning and disinfection station
RKI	Robert-Koch-Institut	Robert Koch Institute
RLT	Raumlufttechnische Anlagen	Technical Equipment for indoor air equipment
RNA	Ribonukleinsäure	Ribonucleic acid
S		
StGB	Strafgesetzbuch	Criminal Code
STIKO	Ständige Impfkommission	Standing Vaccination Commission of RKI
T		
TGEA	Trypton Glucose Extrakt Agar	Trypton Glucose Extract Agar
TI	Technische Information	Technical Information
TNI	Terminale Niereninsuffizienz	Terminal Renal Insufficiency

TRBA	Technische Regeln Biologische Arbeitsstoffe	Technical Regulations for Biological Working Materials
TRGS	Technische Regeln für Gefahrstoffe	Technical Regulations for Hazardous Substances
TrinkwV	Trinkwasser-verordnung	Drinking Water Ordinance
TSE	Transmissible spongioforme Enzephalopathie	Transmissible Spongioform Encephalopathy
TT-Virusinfektion	Transfusion Transmitted Virus Infection	Transfusion Transmitted Virus Infection
TWV	Trinkwasser-verordnung	Drinking Water Ordinance
U		
US	United States	United States
UVV	Unfallverhütungs-vorschriften	Accident Prevention Regulations
V		
VDE	Verband der Elektrotechnik, Elektronik, Informationstechnik	Association for Electrical, Electronic & Information Technologies
W		
WC	Water Closet	Water Closet
Z		
ZfW	Zentrum für Weiterbildung	Centre for Further Education
ZKV	Zentrale Konzentratversorgung	Central concentrate supply
ZVK	Zentralvenöser Katheter	Central venous catheter